P9-AGN-088

PAPERBACK
EXCHANGE
131 Vesta
Reno, Nevada 89502
WE SELL - WE TRADE

DESIGN
YOUR OWN
VITAMIN AND MINERAL
PROGRAM

DESIGN
YOUR OWN
VITAMIN AND
MINERAL PROGRAM

Shari Lieberman, M.A., R.D., and Nancy Bruning

DOUBLEDAY & COMPANY, INC., GARDEN CITY, NEW YORK
1987

Library of Congress Cataloging-in-Publication Data

Lieberman, Shari.
  Design your own vitamin and mineral program.

  Includes index.
  1. Vitamins in human nutrition.   2. Minerals in
human nutrition.   3. Self-care, Health.   I. Bruning,
Nancy.   II. Title.
QP771.L54   1987   613.2'8   86-16200
ISBN 0-385-23309-4
ISBN 0-385-23971-8 (pbk.)

Copyright © 1987 by Shari Lieberman and Nancy Bruning
ALL RIGHTS RESERVED
PRINTED IN THE UNITED STATES OF AMERICA

*This book is dedicated to the memory
of my father, Mort Lieberman*

ACKNOWLEDGMENTS

I would like to thank the following people for their assistance in writing this book: my mother, Sheila, for her loving support; Darwin Buschman, M.D.; Pamela Moss, M.D.; Jeffrey Wolff, M.D.; Michael V. Reitano, M.D.; and Dr. Philip Zimmerman.

CONTENTS

PART THREE: THE MINERALS   113

PART FOUR: APPENDIXES AND NOTES   163

INTRODUCTION BY RONALD L. HOFFMAN, M.D.

It is with great pleasure that I greet the timely publication of *Design Your Own Vitamin and Mineral Program*. The past few years have witnessed an explosion of information in the nutrition field. As recently as 1960, just a handful of academic nutrition journals were in existence; today, worldwide, there are over one hundred. Increasingly, scientists, doctors, professional nutritionists, and laypersons alike are coming to the realization that nutrition can make a difference in our lives.

The new public awareness of nutrition is evidenced by an enormous proliferation of articles, books, and health-oriented TV and radio shows, not to mention health food stores and natural food restaurants. In unprecedented numbers, Americans are changing their diets and taking nutritional supplements.

The results are just beginning to become manifest, but early indications are that this grass-roots movement is helping our nation reclaim its health: Roughly twenty-five years after the cholesterol–heart disease connection began to be publicized, we are experiencing a surprising, sharp decline in the national incidence of heart attack death, the number one killer in the United States. With new awareness about the diet-cancer link and nutritional risk factors for hypertension and diabetes, we will hopefully see a diminution in the death rate from these nutritionally preventable diseases.

Regrettably, the medical profession is missing the opportunity to lead Americans to higher levels of health via nutrition. Frustrated medical consumers are turning away in droves from the drug-oriented approach their physicians too often offer them. Myself a product of a medical education, I am aware of the gross deficiencies in a doctor's exposure to contemporary nutritional issues. Nutrition in medical school is often relegated to a handful of poorly attended lectures. Harried doctors-in-training are too worried about achieving passing marks in "important" courses such as pharmacology to give nutrition much serious consideration. The pressured life-style of medical school soon gives way to the harsh demands of the hospital wards, and coffee, sugary snacks, and fast food become the dietary mainstays of tomorrow's doctors.

Little wonder then that broad segments of the public are turning away from "orthodox" medicine and are embracing a self-care model with nutrition at its core.

But information about nutrition is proliferating at such a fast rate that the average layperson is bewildered by contradictory claims: Which is better—the high-carbohydrate or the high-protein diet? How best can we safeguard immunity? What nutrients counteract cardiovascular disease? And on and on the controversies proliferate.

Into this arena steps a new breed of skilled practitioner—the rigorously scientifically trained nutritionist, of which Shari Lieberman is one of our most outstanding contemporary examples. Nutritionists like her are the "barefoot doctors" of the new Nutrition Revolution. In the absence of sufficient numbers of adequately trained nutritionally oriented physicians, they extend the benefits of their expert training in nutrition to the public. Their numbers are increasing as a measure of the beneficial role they play in response to overwhelming popular demand.

The new nutritionists are every bit as scientifically grounded as their medical peers. Many, like Shari, make use of vast computer data bases to stay abreast of the latest nutritional breakthroughs. They are as comfortable thumbing through *The New England Journal of Medicine* as through the pages of the latest natural foods cookbook. It is through their efforts that the latest discoveries in nutrition are translated to day-to-day dietary prescriptions for an American public hungry for nutritional guidance.

Good books on nutrition are hard to find. They often deal in simplistic formulas, offering panaceas instead of reasoned arguments. The proper balance must be struck between scientific accuracy and ease of presentation—and this is something that Shari Lieberman and her gifted colleague, Nancy Bruning, have achieved admirably in *Design Your Own Vitamin and Mineral Program.* I have confidence in the scholarly and scientific way the two authors have researched their information. I would not hesitate to recommend this book to my physician colleagues as a primer on vitamin supplementation; armed with the information it contains, they would be more likely to intelligently reply to the questions of patients who have already done *their* homework on nutrition.

A new era is dawning in the field of nutrition. We are emerging from a limited definition of proper nutrition as mere absence of deficiency to an awareness that nutrition may open to us new vistas of optimal health.

From the pages of distinguished medical journals to the side panels of high-fiber breakfast cereals, the same message is being loudly proclaimed: *Nutrition Matters!!* And it is with this book that we become better prepared to intelligently heed that clarion call.

PREFACE

Shari Lieberman has done it! She has put together a contemporary and easily applied book that not only documents but also provides step-by-step implementation of nutritional approaches toward improved health and wellness. The field of nutrition is overwhelmed with books by nonqualified individuals. But Ms. Lieberman, as a Registered Dietitian, has woven that very delicate path between the body of hard nutritional science and the nutrition of the future, which makes this book very readable and applicable to the needs of people who are looking for substantive information in the field of nutrition and health promotion.

Ms. Lieberman is not only a student of nutritional science but also a clinician who has dealt with individuals in search of answers as to how to feel better. This book provides that rare blend of information that should prove useful to any reader who is looking for methods of instituting their own health responsibility program.

Jeffrey S. Bland, Ph.D.
President, J.S.B. & Associates Inc.
Director, Linus Pauling Institute

WHAT'S YOUR
VITAMIN IQ?

1. Vitamin E has been shown to:

    A. Improve your sex life

    B. Help prevent cancer

    C. Prevent baldness

    D. None of the above

2. Enriched white bread is just as nutritious as whole wheat bread.

    A. True

    B. False

3. Which drug(s) increase your need for certain vitamins and/or minerals?

    A. Antibiotics

    B. Aspirin

    C. Birth control pills

    D. All of the above

4. Who generally requires a higher intake of vitamins and minerals?

    A. Senior citizens

    B. Body builders

    C. Marathon runners

    D. All of the above

5. Which mineral(s) have been shown to protect against many forms of cancer?

    A. Calcium

    B. Magnesium

    C. Selenium

    D. None of the above

6. When is the best time to take supplements?

    A. In the morning

    B. In the evening

    C. With meals

    D. On an empty stomach

7. As long as you take supplements, you can eat whatever you want.

    A. True

    B. False

8. Vitamin C has been shown to _____ colds.

    A. Cure

    B. Prevent

    C. Shorten the duration of

    D. All of the above

9. Which nutrient(s) may be effective in preventing cardiovascular disease?

    A. Calcium

    B. Vitamin E

    C. Niacin

    D. All of the above

10. The more supplements you take, the better.

    A. True

    B. False

ANSWERS

1. **B.** Many studies have shown that vitamin E helps protect us against the harmful effects of a variety of carcinogens and toxins, including carbon tetrachloride, mercury, lead, benzene, ozone, and nitrous oxide. It prevents the formation of potent carcinogens called nitrosamines from the nitrates found in air pollution, cigarette smoke, and some foods. Vitamin E also prevents vitamins A and C, two other vitamins which protect us from carcinogens, from losing their potency in the body. Although severe vitamin E deficiency did cause infertility in experimental animals, no studies have shown this nutrient to improve the sex life of humans. Vitamin E does not prevent baldness. (See Chapter 8.)

2. **B.** The flour used to make white bread has been depleted of *over twenty* nutrients, including up to 50 percent of the vitamin C, 85 percent of the vitamin B-6, and 72 percent of the zinc. The manufacturers then put back a handful of these nutrients (five, to be exact), and calls the end result "enriched"! Whole wheat bread is much higher in almost every vitamin and mineral, including trace minerals such as chromium, selenium, and manganese; it is also higher in protein and fiber. (See Chapter 2.)

3. **D.** It is widely recognized that many drugs interact with nutrients in the body, often causing depletion. Antibiotics have been shown to interfere with the B vitamins, vitamin C, and calcium. They may also destroy useful bacteria in the colon, thus hindering vitamin K synthesis. Estrogen-containing medications such as birth control pills deplete the body of vitamin B-6, folic acid, and vitamin C. Even aspirin, if used over a long period of time, may deplete vitamin C and folic acid. (See Chapter 2.)

4. **D.** Marathoners and body builders, because of their exercise regimens, are under physical stress and this increases their need for many vitamins and minerals. In addition, people who exercise heavily tend to eat large amounts of carbohydrates, which increases the need for thiamin. Finally, sweating has been shown to increase the excretion of certain essential nutrients. Many studies have shown that the elderly are also at high risk of low levels of nutrients, especially calcium; vitamins B-6, B-12, E, and D; folic acid; and zinc, because of reduced absorption and poor eating habits. (See Chapter 2.)

5. C. There is a higher incidence of cancer among people who live in geographical areas where the soil is lower in this mineral. Studies have correlated many forms of cancer, but especially breast cancer, with a low selenium intake. There is some evidence that calcium may protect against colon cancer, but the data is too preliminary to draw any firm conclusions. (See Chapter 29.)

6. C. Vitamin and mineral supplements are best absorbed if taken along with food. It is even better if doses are divided throughout the day. Although some people believe it is advantageous to take certain nutrients in the morning and others in the evening, there is no evidence that this is anything but theory at this point. (See Chapter 4.)

7. B. Supplements are just that—*supplements* to be taken in addition to an intelligent diet, in order to make up for the nutrients lost in our food owing to many factors including shipping, storage, and processing. Supplements are not meant to overcome a diet that is too high in fat and sugar and too low in fiber. They are part of a total health program that should include good fresh food, exercise, stress reduction, and avoidance of substances known to be harmful to the body. (See Chapter 5.)

8. C. Vitamin C has been shown to shorten the duration of colds and lessen the severity of the symptoms. Vitamin C is an important component of the immune system, but has never been conclusively proven to either prevent or cure the common cold. (See Chapter 20.)

9. D. Many studies correlate a higher calcium intake with lower blood pressure. Vitamin E may reduce cholesterol in the blood, and increase HDL (high-density lipoproteins) levels (the "good" type of cholesterol). It may also help prevent platelets from clogging the arteries. Niacin has been shown to be effective in reducing cholesterol and triglycerides in the blood. In fact, two studies recommend niacin as the treatment of choice for these conditions. (See Chapters 8, 13, and 21.)

10. B. There is an optimum amount of each nutrient for each individual, beyond which the benefits are small or nonexistent. There is no reason to take, for example, 150 milligrams of the B vitamins when 50 milligrams will do the job for you. Although even very high doses of vitamin and mineral supplements are generally not harmful, it makes no sense economically or healthwise to take more than you really need. (See Chapter 4.)

Your Score:

7–10 Correct . . . . Excellent

4–6 Correct . . . . Average

0–3 Correct . . . . Poor

THE PURPOSE OF
THIS BOOK

My becoming a dietitian/nutritionist—as well as my writing this book—came about in a rather roundabout way. Initially, I wanted to be a medical doctor. I was interested in science and I wanted to work with people, to help them. I thought being a physician would allow me to do this.

However, as a pre-med student, I learned that traditional Western medicine takes quite a rigid and fragmented approach. It is primarily concerned with treating isolated symptoms and diseases, rather than promoting the health of the whole person. I realized that although conventional medicine has its place and can do a lot of good—even perform miracles—that prevention is a far more potent tool in the larger scheme of things. In addition, it became clear to me that nutrition should be our first line of defense if an illness or condition is not life-threatening. Compared to modern Western medicine, the nutritional approach is a safe, nontoxic, effective alternative.

My interest in nutrition was originally piqued at the age of fourteen, when I came down with mononucleosis. An avid tennis player, I was crushed when my doctor told me I would need three months of bedrest in order to recover. However, my father started me on a program of vitamin A and C supplements. Imagine my physician's surprise when I returned to my tennis two weeks later! As I continued to take supplements, I noticed that not only was I free of colds, but I felt absolutely great.

As I grew older, another compelling reason to explore the potential impact of nutrition took shape. I discovered I had a hereditary predisposition to heart disease. It seemed everybody in my family was dying of heart disease at a relatively early age: Both my grandfathers had heart attacks, my mother's mother died of a stroke, my father's two brothers had heart problems, and my own father died of a heart attack at the age of fifty-nine. There I was, at the age of twenty-two, with a cholesterol count of 225, and HDLs of 46. Conventional medicine considered these levels acceptable. But my research of the medical literature showed that this was an overly complacent attitude. Some researchers were saying that cholesterol levels higher than 200 in people under forty years of age increased the risk of heart disease.

Although the research then was new and sketchy, an alarm went off somewhere inside me. Was I doomed to watch my cholesterol gradually climb up and up while I stood idly by? Was my future to consist of toxic drug therapy in an attempt to control my cholesterol which had zoomed sky-high? There was also some research showing that simple dietary changes, certain supplements, and regular aerobic exercise would make a difference. Although this research was also new and controversial, I decided to take action. My cholesterol is now down to 185, and my HDLs up to 96. As a result, I now have a much lower risk of heart disease. I am happy to report that I have had similar results with my patients.

My coauthor, Nancy Bruning, also came to nutrition and the writing of this book because of a very personal concern and involvement. A patient of mine had told her I work with cancer patients who are undergoing chemotherapy, and we met when she interviewed me for her book, *Coping with Chemotherapy*. A former cancer chemotherapy patient herself, she was primarily interested in researching therapies that could be used to complement conventional chemotherapy to make it more comfortable, less damaging, and perhaps more effective. Although she learned firsthand the important role that nutrition plays in such circumstances, she too realized that disease prevention is a superior tactic and that nutrition can have a tremendous impact on overall health. Six years post diagnosis, in excellent health and her chemotherapy book completed, she decided to concentrate her energies on writing about disease prevention.

My research and clinical experience in working with a wide variety of people have shown me that in today's world, most people do not get all the vitamins and minerals they need from food. As a result, they do not enjoy optimum health and they are setting the stage for poor health in the future. Vitamin and mineral supplements may be our best protection against this. But vitamin and mineral supplementation is an individual matter. Up to now it has been difficult, if not impossible, for the average person to determine what he or she should take. My purpose in writing this book is to provide you with information in a form that you will be able to use to actually create your own individual vitamin and mineral program.

According to a 1985 FDA-funded survey, almost 40 percent of the American population is taking one or more supplements. But do people know what to take, or why they are taking it? My contact with people as a private clinician, as a teacher, and as a lecturer has taught me that people want to individualize and optimize their vitamin regimens to suit their own lives, in much the same way they want to individualize and optimize their workouts and their diets.

As a registered dietitian and nutritionist, I see fifty people in my office every week. They come to me with a variety of problems and needs. Some are specific, such as acne, psoriasis, thinning hair, menstrual problems, blood sugar problems, intestinal disorders, high blood pressure, high cholesterol, an inability to sleep, fatigue, depression, or nervousness. These people turn to nutrition as an adjunct or an alternative to the treatment offered by their physicians. But most people who come to me are not obviously sick—they are interested in nutrition as a means of improving their health and preventing illness. They want to live longer, healthier lives, to feel better, look better, have more energy, withstand stress better, and be able to avoid or minimize diseases that range from the common cold to cancer.

They come to me because they are very confused about vitamin supplementation. In spite of all the books and articles they've read, they still don't know how to apply all the available information to their own lives. Nutrition is a very complex subject, challenging for even the qualified professional to understand in all its subtleties. The field is growing, and becoming full of self-styled experts who bombard you with contradictory advice and information almost daily. You, the public, are in the unfortunate position of being caught in the crossfire. Many people solve this problem by going to a "personal nutritionist." However, progressive nutritionists are not available to everyone. This book was written for people who are seeing a nutritionist as well as for those who are not. It is also a useful tool for practitioners who are not trained in nutrition and are interested in learning about the progressive approach to this subject.

Today, people say they either "believe" in taking vitamins, or they don't, as if this were some kind of religion, based on blind faith. I want to reassure you that the progressive nutritional approach to health is not a religion. It is an emerging science that is taking its rightful place next to other health sciences. This poses two basic problems that I have written this book to correct:

The first is that because it is a science, the language can get very technical. My education and interpersonal experience have taught me how to translate highly technical data into a language that the average person can understand.

The second is that because it is a new science, some of the information is less available or incomplete. In writing this book I have researched the most up-to-date professional journals, including foreign research journals. I have interpreted them and synthesized the information to provide you with the most comprehensive, unified, and scientifically sound picture of what vitamins and minerals can—and cannot—do for you.

As you will see in this book, people are not getting the government-established Recommended Daily Allowances (RDAs) from their diets. In addition, the RDAs are not high enough for many people. *Design Your Own Vitamin and Mineral Program* acknowledges the redefinition of health as not just the absence of disease, but *optimum* physical and mental well-being. This book is written from the viewpoint that amounts in excess of the RDAs can be preventive, therapeutic, and safe. I have called these excess amounts the Optimum Daily Allowance (ODA)—a dosage range within which nearly everyone can find his or her individual amount. Every recommendation in *Design Your Own Vitamin and Mineral Program* is based on the latest reliable scientific data including studies published in well-respected professional journals as well as on my successes with patients, not on hearsay or on highly questionable studies. I make it clear when contradictory or inconclusive data exist that further studies are needed. For example, I would be delighted to be able to say that large doses of vitamin C cure cancer, but the evidence so far has not supported this statement. On the other hand, the evidence is strong enough to recommend taking vitamin C as a *preventive measure* against certain cancers.

Nutritionists, physicians, and researchers are in agreement that vitamins and minerals are essential for human health. They differ only as far as specific uses and amounts are concerned. Clearly, some of the claims for "megavitamins" are less well supported than others. As a result, people are taking the wrong vitamins and minerals, in the wrong amounts, for the wrong reasons. Many of them are wasting their time and money, either on multivitamins, which can be hit-or-miss, or on dosages which are either unnecessarily high or too low to have an appreciable effect. Many people would like to take supplements, but are confused and so have given up or don't know how to begin.

If you, like many of my patients, have looked through or read other nutrition books but found them too technical, filled with too much or unnecessary information, or not specific enough, this book is for you. *Design Your Own Vitamin and Mineral Program* will clear the air. This book deals only with vitamin and mineral supplements generally available to the public. This does not mean that you are getting *less* information, just *less distracting* information. You get clarity, not clutter. I present the information in a straightforward, usable form. It takes the confusion out of taking supplements, and gives you—in simple, honest, realistic terms— exactly the foundation you need to create a workable vitamin/mineral plan for yourself.

Part One explains the RDAs and the ODAs as well as how to use the book. These introductory chapters give you a basic grasp of the concepts, goals, and guidelines of vitamin and mineral supplementation.

Part Two consists of individual chapters on each vitamin, including the doses I recommend to my patients for general optimum health and for specific problems.

Part Three consists of individual chapters on minerals.

Part Four provides handy reference charts and sample worksheets to help you apply what you have learned and custom-design an individual vitamin and mineral program. I have also included reference abstracts for each vitamin and mineral chapter—summaries of the most recent scientific studies for anyone who wishes to research the subject further.

PART ONE

Chapter 1

WHAT ARE VITAMINS AND MINERALS?

Vitamins and minerals are nutrients that are essential to life. They are so-called "micronutrients" because, in comparison to the other nutrients—carbohydrates, proteins, fats, and water—we need them in relatively small amounts.

Vitamins function by and large as *coenzymes*. Enzymes are catalysts or activators in the chemical reactions that are continually taking place in our bodies. Vitamins are a fundamental part of the enzymes, the way your muscles are a fundamental part of your arms and legs. Most people are aware that we have enzymes to help us digest our food. But enzymes do more than help us digest food. They are at the very foundation of *all* our bodily functions. Enzymes are what make things happen, and happen faster.

Without enzymes, you can't breathe, blink, or walk. Your body can't break down proteins into essential amino acids, electrons can't flow, and nerve transmissions can't occur. You wouldn't be able to pull your hand out of the fire (or put it there in the first place), smell a rose, see the sunset, or taste an apple. For example, a particular enzyme which requires vitamin B-6 to be activated is needed to transmit nerve impulses to your fingers. No matter how plentiful this enzyme is in your body, if you are deficient in B-6, this enzyme will not be activated. As a result you might feel some numbness in your fingers.

Minerals, many of which also function as coenzymes, are needed for the proper composition of our body fluids, in blood and bone formation, and to maintain healthy nerve function.

In addition to their role as coenzymes, some micronutrients have other functions. For example, vitamin E acts as an antioxidant (see Chapter 8); calcium, magnesium, and phosphorus form our bones; and active vitamin D functions as a hormone.

After they have been absorbed, vitamins and minerals actually become a part of the structure of the body—of the cells, enzymes, hormones, muscles, blood, and bone. They become a part of the "body pool" and as such stay in the body for varying amounts of time. They can be utilized immediately, or stored and utilized over a period of time.

The vitamins that stay in the body for a short period of time—two to four days—are called *water-soluble vitamins.* The B vitamins and vitamin C belong to this group. Water-soluble vitamins begin to be utilized by the body from the minute they are absorbed through your digestive system and must be replenished regularly. Since they are not stored, but quickly excreted from the body, toxicities are virtually unknown.

Fat-soluble vitamins, on the other hand, stay in the body for a longer period of time. Vitamins A, D, E, and K belong to this group. They are usually stored in fat (lipid) tissue, but some may also be stored in some organs, especially the liver. Therefore, you can have toxicity problems with some of the fat-soluble vitamins, but only when you take very large doses.

Minerals also belong to two groups: the "macro" or bulk minerals and the "micro" or trace minerals. Macro minerals are needed in larger amounts than the micro minerals. The macro minerals include calcium, magnesium, and phosphorus. The micro minerals include zinc, iron, copper, manganese, chromium, selenium, iodine, and potassium. Minerals are stored in various parts of the body—primarily in bone and muscle tissue. Therefore, it is also possible to overdose on minerals if you take extremely large doses.

However, you must remember that there is no vitamin or mineral that is as toxic as most of the drugs you can buy over the counter, including aspirin. In order to reach toxicity, you must go out of your way to abuse supplements by taking massive quantities, usually for a prolonged period of time. The dose ranges I give for vitamins and minerals are completely safe and have never caused any problems in any of my patients.

Chapter 2

THE RDAs—
THE MINIMUM WAGES
OF NUTRITION

Clearly, vitamins and minerals are essential to good health and to life itself. But how do we know whether we are getting enough to ensure good health? For more than forty years, the Recommended Daily Allowances (RDAs) have been our guidelines. They are the U.S. Food and Nutrition Board's estimates of the amounts of nutrients required by most people to prevent overt deficiency symptoms. Much of what you hear about how "we can get everything we need from a well-balanced diet" and "vitamin and mineral supplements are a waste of money" is based on the widespread acceptance of these guidelines. However, while the RDAs were a significant first step in understanding nutrition, we are beginning to realize that they have very important limitations.

Since their inception, the RDAs have been periodically reevaluated and updated based on a continuing analysis of our rapidly expanding knowledge in the area of nutrition. But in 1985, there was such widespread disagreement among the scientists involved that the National Research Council was unable to issue its scheduled new edition of the RDAs. This inability of even the most conservative nutrition experts to agree reflects and illustrates some of the reservations about the RDAs that I and other nutrition clinicians and researchers have been expressing for some time. There are three basic problems I have with the RDAs: (1) You cannot get all the nutrients you need from today's food; (2) The RDAs are not really designed for the individual; and (3) They do not ensure optimum health.

Problem 1: Can You Really Get Everything You Need from Food?

The RDAs are intended to be met solely through the diet. However, it is virtually *impossible* to meet the RDAs from eating the food available to us today. As a clinician who sees real people everyday, I know how impractical and misleading the typical well-balanced diet given in nutrition handbooks can be. Such a diet does not take into consideration people's individual lifestyles, food preferences, and habits; food availability; the inaccuracy of the food value tables; or the loss of nutrients that occurs during storage, shipping, processing, and cooking.

The Myth of the Well-Balanced Diet. In the first place, most people simply do not eat a well-balanced diet, which, according to the latest recommendations of the National Research Council, consists of approximately 30 percent fat, 20 percent protein, 35 percent complex carbohydrates (grains, breads, starchy vegetables), and 15 percent simple carbohydrates (high-sugar foods such as sweets and fruits). Does a frazzled executive take the time to calculate her fat intake? Does an overworked teacher know how much complex carbohydrate he has eaten? Does a teenager or a senior citizen know how much protein is in a cheese danish? Does even the most health-conscious marathon runner eat a perfect diet every day? Of course not.

In addition, there is the calorie problem. A diet that satisfies the RDAs is based on approximately 2000 calories for women, and 3000 calories for men. This is about twice as much as is allowed on the average reducing diet, and it has been estimated that one-third of America is dieting at any one time. Even if we are not dieting, most of us could not consume this many calories and still maintain a desirable weight. If we are dieting, the news is even worse: Researchers found that of eleven published diet-plan books (the F-plan, Scarsdale, Pritikin, Richard Simmons, Atkins, Stillman, I Love New York, I Love America, Beverly Hills, Carbohydrate Craver's, and California diets), *none* provided a full 100 percent of the RDA for thirteen vitamins and minerals.

The danger of large-scale deficiencies is not just theory. I have seen many published reports in the United States, Great Britain, and Europe showing that portions of even affluent societies may be highly deficient in certain nutrients. Women are especially at risk for deficiencies. For example, an American study found that women generally consume 60 percent as many calories as men, and therefore obtain about 60 percent as much of each nutrient as men.

I have found it especially interesting (and frankly, amusing) that a survey of over six hundred dietitians found that nearly 60 percent of them used nutritional supplements. Presumably, a majority of the food experts who have traditionally espoused the view that a balanced diet provides all the nutrients you need now realize how unrealistic this view is.

The Case of the Missing Nutrients. In addition, new evidence shows that the food tables which supposedly tell us the nutrient content of the foods we eat probably overstate the nutrient content of foods. As a result, the orange you just bought is probably not nearly as full of vitamin C as the tables would lead you to believe.

What's more, the nutrient content of foods, especially of minerals, fluctuates widely depending upon the growing conditions. Our soil is depleted of selenium in most parts of the country, and often only marginal levels of zinc, magnesium, calcium, and other minerals exist, too. There is absolutely no guarantee that the soil in which our food is being grown is adequate in these essential minerals.

Fruits and vegetables begin to lose nutrients from the moment they are picked. The food we buy has oftentimes been stored for weeks or months. Most of the "fresh" fruits and vegetables we are eating follow this progression: They are picked, then stored, then shipped, then stored. After we buy them, we store them some more. Then we may cook them, or at least cut or slice them. Or a food may be processed before we buy it. All of these cause further nutrient loss.

For example, the vitamin C content in apples may fall by two-thirds after only two to three months. Potatoes may have 30 milligrams of vitamin C per 100 grams when they are freshly harvested in the fall; but by springtime they have only 8 milligrams per 100 grams, and by summer they have practically none. Green vegetables suffer even more—they lose almost all their vitamin C after a few days of being stored at room temperature. Everyone "knows" that orange juice is high in vitamin C. But few people realize that an orange loses 30 percent of its vitamin C soon after it is squeezed. Commercial orange juice has almost no natural vitamin C left.

Few people realize that a surprising amount of the total nutrient content in many foods exists in a form that is not bioavailable, meaning our bodies can't absorb and use it. About 40 percent of the vitamin C that is left in fresh squeezed orange juice is biologically inactive. According to the food value tables, one cup of green cabbage has 33 milligrams of vitamin C—over half the RDA. What the food table doesn't tell you is that it is present in a form of vitamin C that is very poorly absorbed.

Next, we must consider how the heat, light, water, and chemicals used to process foods further deplete their nutrients. Blanching, which vegetables undergo before they are canned or frozen, can destroy up to 60 percent of the vitamin C content, 40 percent of the riboflavin, and 30 percent of the thiamin. The sterilization process used in canned foods further destroys vitamins: for example, 39 percent of the vitamin A may be destroyed, and 69 percent of the remaining thiamin. While freezing itself seems preferable to canning, vitamin C may be depleted by about 25 percent. After they are processed, foods are stored and continue to lose their nutrients.

The simple act of cutting fruits and vegetables will encourage both vitamin and mineral losses. Cooking methods generally deplete about 50 percent of the less stable vitamins, especially vitamin C. This includes not just vegetables, but meat, which may lose up to half of its thiamin, B-6, and pantothenic acid during cooking. By the time you put cooked peas on the table, there may be only 44 percent of the original vitamin C (for fresh peas), 17 percent (for frozen peas), or as little as 6 percent (for canned peas).

Perhaps one of the greatest injustices inflicted upon foods occurs during the milling of grains: When wheat is processed into white flour, up to 40 percent of the vitamin C and from 65 to 85 percent of various B vitamins are depleted. In addition, many minerals are lost, including 59 percent of the magnesium and 72 percent of the zinc. You also lose significant amounts of other vitamins, protein, and fiber. All in all, an appalling twenty-six essential nutrients are removed. The food industry then puts back a few cents' worth of iron, calcium, niacin, thiamin, and riboflavin—and calls their bread "enriched"!

Problem 2: Are the RDAs Really for Everyone?

The RDAs are "one size fits all." The RDAs are designed to satisfy the needs of a mythical "average healthy person," not the individual. Unfortunately, this person does not exist in reality, just as the average American family, with its 2.2 children, never really existed. You are as different from me as I am from Telly Savalas. There are twenty-five documented inborn errors of metabolism, some of which can increase an individual's vitamin requirements by a factor of 10 to 1000. These have overt symptoms and include Cooley's anemia (iron) and Wilson's disease (copper). Experiments have shown that it is highly probable that many individuals may have difficulties with specific nutrients on a more subtle scale which may not be so easily diagnosed. These may, however, diminish our quality of life and be implicated in future problems as serious as cancer and, as we have seen in my case, heart disease. Not only do we all come into this world with our own individual biological blueprint, but we continue to change and undergo different experiences, such as environmental pollution, stress, disease, drug therapy, and aging. Each of these has the potential for increasing our needs and/or interfering with the metabolism of nutrients.

Environmental Pollution. Today there are an unprecedented number of chemicals all around us—in our food, our water, the very air we breathe. The Environmental Protection Association has estimated that sixty thousand chemicals have been buried or dumped over the years, and are now penetrating our water supply. Automobiles and industry spew millions of pounds of pollutants into the atmosphere every year. Our food has become a chemical feast that is sprayed with pesticides, injected with hormones, fed with antibiotics, and adulterated with over three thousand chemicals in the form of artificial colors, flavors, textures, and preservatives. Cigarette smokers not only pollute their own lungs, but endanger the health of others through secondhand smoke. Living and/or working with smokers can be equivalent to smoking several cigarettes a day. Many of these chemicals are definitely, and others are potentially, hazardous to human health.

However, it has been found that certain vitamins and minerals are protective against some of these toxic substances. For example, vitamins C and E have been shown to be protective against nitrosamine, a carcinogen your body forms from the nitrates and nitrites found in processed meat such as hot dogs, bacon, ham, and bologna. These same carcinogens will form from pollutants in the air and in cigarette smoke. I give vitamins A and E to my patients who live in large cities, especially if they are foolish enough to smoke. I give vitamin A or beta-carotene because it must be protective, too, since so many studies link higher levels of this vitamin with a lower incidence of many types of cancer. Toxic chemicals have become a prime suspect in male infertility: Sperm counts in the United

States have declined by 80 percent over the last fifty years. But vitamin C has been shown to increase the percentage of normal sperm, sperm motility, and sperm viability in infertile men with lowered sperm count. Whether the chemicals deplete nutrients or increase your requirements, I feel it's wise to superfortify our bodies to withstand these chemical insults.

Stress. It has been well documented that if you are under any sort of stress that you deplete your store of vitamins and minerals more rapidly. Whether they are physical, such as strenuous exercise, or emotional, such as changing jobs, stressful situations generally call for higher intakes of vitamins and minerals.

Disease/Disorders. There are many diseases that interfere with the ingestion, digestion, absorption, and requirement of nutrients. Diseases that affect the digestive system such as celiac disease, Crohn's disease, irritable bowel syndrome, lactose intolerance, and bacterial, viral, and parasitic infections are the most obvious. But infections in *any* part of the body also rapidly deplete the body of most vitamins and minerals. In addition, your appetite usually decreases during times of illness, which further depletes your nutrient stores. During the recuperation process following an illness, trauma, burns, or surgery, the body's stores of nutrients need to be replenished and the injured tissues repaired. Nutrients are also important for building up our immune systems, especially at critical times. Ironically, a downward spiral often occurs, in which illness depletes the body of nutrients, which lowers the resistance to infections, which in turn lowers the nutrient level even more, and so on. The results of several studies have indicated that hospital patients as a group are some of the most malnourished people in the world. One study showed that only 12 percent of the patients studied had normal levels of vitamins in their bodies. Yet most of them had been eating a "normal American diet."

As you will see in the upcoming chapters on the individual vitamins and minerals, people with overt, diagnosed medical conditions or diseases often have low levels of one or more vitamins or minerals in their bodies. This occurs even though these conditions are not usually associated with nutritional deficiencies. This may indicate that nutrient deficiencies do play a previously unacknowledged role in the development of a particular disease or condition. Or it may mean that deficiencies are a direct or indirect result of the condition. In any event, I always take into consideration my patient's present and past physical condition, as well as their family's health history, when giving them supplements.

Drugs/Medication. It is widely recognized that many drugs interact with nutrients in the body, often causing depletion. Many antibiotics are known to interfere with the B-complex vitamins. Hormones in medications such as oral contraceptives appear to reduce the levels of some of the water-soluble vitamins. Antacids, which coat the walls of the intestines to protect from stomach acid, also prevent several nutrients from being absorbed. Questran, a commonly prescribed drug used to lower cholesterol, limits the absorption of vitamins A, D, E, and K. Tetracycline, a widely used antibiotic, interferes with the absorption of calcium.

Alcoholics have multiple nutritional deficiencies, owing to many factors, which include alcohol's being used as a substitute for food and alcohol's interfering with the absorption of nutrients.

Aging. Studies have shown that your body changes throughout life. As you age, your organs generally tend to function less efficiently. Your digestion may be affected in several ways. Absorption and utilization of nutrients are decreased. As your level of physical activity diminishes and your metabolism slows, your overall food intake goes down too, putting the elderly at particular risk for suboptimal nutrition.

There have been many studies done on older people showing that they are simply not getting enough nutrients from their diets. It may come as no surprise to hear that a survey of fourteen nursing homes found that not one of them provided meals that met the RDAs for all nutrients. Another study, of 270 healthy people who lived in the area of Albuquerque, New Mexico, is startling. They were Caucasian, were highly educated, had higher than average incomes, and were considered to be "health conscious." Yet the study found that up to 86 percent of the women and 85 percent of the men were getting less than the RDAs for vitamins B-6, B-12, E, D, folic acid, calcium, and zinc. As we age, we do require more nutrients—particularly calcium and magnesium. In addition, many diseases associated with aging, such as cancer, high blood pressure, heart disease, and diabetes, have recently been shown to have nutritional implications.

Problem 3: Do the RDAs Ensure Optimum Health?

The RDAs are designed to prevent only overt deficiency symptoms. Prolonged deficiency in a certain vitamin or mineral will generally result in severe disease with easily observable symptoms. For example, vitamin A deficiency will lead to night blindness and other eye problems; niacin deficiency will cause pellagra characterized by "diarrhea, dermatitis, and dementia"; iron or B-12 deficiency will result in anemia. There is no question that the estimated RDAs are sufficient to prevent severe deficiency disease in most people. But are they enough to maintain optimum health? Is looking at severe, overt deficiency symptoms an accurate way of determining what you need? What about everything that has happened in the body up until that point? Maybe there are subtle changes that occur in the cells before the body manifests itself in overt deficiency symptoms such as skin sores, mental disturbances, crippling bone loss, or debilitating nervous system problems. Chapter 3 is devoted to this issue and explains how the alternative to the RDA, the ODA, may help to ensure *optimal* health, not just absence of disease.

As it currently stands, the RDA is a limited, outmoded concept, the meaning and usefulness of which is being questioned even by the experts who are responsible for establishing and maintaining it. In today's world, the RDAs are the nutritional equivalent of the minimum wage. Yes, they are probably enough to keep you alive, but how good is the quality of that life? And why should you not strive for something better?

THE CAVEMAN DIET

Some researchers have argued that the best diet for us is one that resembles the diet our remote ancestors consumed. Our genetic constitution has changed very little since modern human beings appeared about forty thousand years ago. One of the factors that played a part in influencing our genetic makeup was the food that was available at that time. It stands to reason that one logical approach to estimating our needs would be to look at what our early ancestors actually ate. The fact that "cavemen" may have died at an early age is beside the point—they lived a much more precarious existence than we did. The point is that these are the people who were able to survive at all—at least until they were old enough to reproduce and pass on their genes. In a study published in *The New England Journal of Medicine,* the authors found that Paleolithic nutrition differed significantly from ours. Among other findings, they concluded that from their diet of 35 percent animal food and 65 percent plant foods such as fruits and vegetables, our early ancestors took in 1579 milligrams calcium (the RDA is 800 milligrams), and nearly 400 milligrams vitamin C per day (the RDA is 60 milligrams). They also probably obtained much higher amounts of the B vitamins than the current RDA recommends.

Among the "primitive" hunter-gatherer people of today, whose way of eating most closely resembles those of our ancestors, the so-called diseases of civilization (coronary heart disease, hypertension, diabetes, and some types of cancer) are virtually unknown—even in the elderly. It is generally agreed that our present diet—high-fat, low-fiber—plays a role in the epidemic of these diseases. This same type of diet is also lower in certain vitamins and minerals. We have already seen a change from the old dietary guidelines to a lower-fat, higher-fiber diet which is considered to be optimal and preventive. It is my hope that the RDAs for vitamins and minerals will one day be approached from this same viewpoint.

Chapter 3

THE OPTIMUM DAILY ALLOWANCES (ODAs)

Recent evidence indicates that the RDAs are far too low because vitamins and minerals do more than just prevent the severe, overt symptoms that are traditionally associated with deficiencies. Remember: *Vitamins and minerals are used in every process of the body.* We now know, for example, that vitamin A does more than prevent night blindness, that thiamin prevents more than beriberi, and that vitamin C certainly does much more than prevent scurvy.

SUBCLINICAL DEFICIENCIES

State-of-the-art biochemistry shows that these classical, overt deficiency symptoms are merely the last event in a long chain of reactions in the body, the way an erupting volcano or earthquake is the last dramatic step in processes that occur underground. That we are not always aware of these processes does not mean that they do not exist, or that they will not eventually cause an explosion of ill health at some point in the future. When we do not get enough of a specific vitamin, the initial reactions occur on the molecular level. The first thing that happens is a depletion of the vitamin stores in the body. Then, the enzymes of which the vitamin is a part become depleted. This in turn brings about changes on the cellular level: Some of the cells of the body, which depend upon these enzymes, can no longer carry out their normal functions. It is not until the depletion is prolonged and severe that the classical clinical signs of deficiency appear.

Such cellular changes are also known as *subclinical deficiencies* because they are not the kind of deficiencies that your doctor could necessarily discover through a routine physical exam and blood tests. Although they may not be obvious, easily definable, or immediately debilitating, they may cause minor problems now, and major problems later on. Studies have shown that although these subclinical signs are subtle, they *do* have an effect on the body's well-being. For example, volunteers who were depleted of vitamin B-1 showed no detectable changes in the body for the first five to ten days. After ten days, there was evidence of changes in the cells' metabolism. Classical anatomical signs of B-1 deficiency became obvious only after about two hundred days. However, during that time, the subjects experienced a gradual decline in their health with nonspecific symptoms of loss of weight, loss of appetite, general malaise, insomnia, and irritability.

The subtle, subclinical changes due to poor nutrition may be responsible for a broad range of diffuse, nonspecific conditions that can at first be merely annoying and reduce our overall health and quality of life. They are often related to stress, aging, and a failing immune system. They can include chronic fatigue, skin problems, recurrent or lingering infections and colds, digestive problems, sleep problems, headaches, hormonal problems, depression, and nervousness. They may also set up conditions in the body that leave us more vulnerable to genetically predisposed diseases and conditions such as cardiovascular disease, diabetes, and cancer. The role that the other nutrients such as fat and carbohydrates play in these diseases is becoming more and more solidly documented. Why should we be surprised at the accumulating evidence that vitamins and minerals also play a part?

NUTRITION—NATURE'S PROTECTOR

Our *immune system* is a complex interaction of blood cells and special proteins acting together to defend us from harm. Improving the immune response is the main thrust behind modern preventive medicine because it protects us in so many important ways. For example, the immune system has the ability to engulf and kill bacteria and viruses; it can also repair or destroy a damaged cell before it grows into a cancerous tumor. This system, though powerful, is extremely delicate, its parts exquisitely interdependent upon one another. If any one aspect is compromised, we may become more susceptible to infections, degenerative diseases including cancer and diabetes, and perhaps cardiovascular disease and certain forms of arthritis.

Inadequate nutrition has been shown in many studies to weaken one or more of the components of our defense system. Inadequate protein, low fiber, and a high-fat diet have all been implicated in impaired immunity. In addition, vitamins and minerals play integral roles. Excesses of the RDAs of almost all vitamins and minerals have been shown to enhance immunity. Those which seem to exert the most profound effect are vitamins A, B-6, pantothenic acid, riboflavin, folic acid, B-12, C, E, selenium, zinc, iron, and magnesium.

Our defense system not only fights bacteria and viruses, but also protects us from *free radicals*. Free radicals, including peroxides, are by-products formed in our bodies when molecules of fat react with oxygen. This is a process that is similar to that which occurs when cooking fats become rancid. Oxidation has also been compared to the formation of rust. Free radicals are very irritating to our cells and can upset their delicate processes. This cell damage can accumulate over time and has been associated with the signs of aging and serious degenerative disease such as arthritis, hardening of the arteries, and heart and kidney ailments. Free radicals are also thought to contribute to the development of cancer.

Free radicals are formed by exposure to toxic chemicals in our food, water, and air; radiation; excessive sunlight; and also in part by normal bodily processes including the metabolization of polyunsaturated fats. Their formation is going on all the time, but our body has certain defense mechanisms that keep these processes under control. One way is by repairing the cell damage they cause. Another way is to intercept the free radicals before they do any harm. There are certain nutrients including vitamins A, C and E and selenium which are called *antioxidants* because they help the body protect itself in this way, or are protective themselves. For example, a wide variety of enzymes, which require certain vitamins and minerals, are used to stop the oxidation process. One of these, gluta-thione peroxidase, requires selenium; another, superoxide dismutase, requires manganese and zinc. In one study, vitamin C (200 milligrams twice a day) reduced the lipid (fat) peroxide level by 13 percent in one year; vitamins E and C together reduced the levels by 25 percent. Vitamin E works synergistically with selenium and is known as a "scavenger" of free radicals formed by the oxidation of fats. It also protects vitamins A and C from oxidation, thus preserving the potency of these other two antioxidants.

If our bodies become overwhelmed by free radicals, and/or if we are not getting enough of the protective vitamins and minerals from our diets (which we are not), taking supplements can help protect us. For example, vegetable oils are being consumed in greater quantity because of the ability of their polyunsaturated fatty acids (PUFA) to reduce cholesterol. Vegetable oils are naturally high in vitamin E; however, the heat used to process commercial oils destroys their vitamin E. Since vitamin E prevents the oxidation of PUFA, I feel supplementation of vitamin E is necessary. Another example is selenium, a mineral which is generally depleted from our soil. Low intakes of selenium have been implicated in many forms of cancer. The RDA of vitamin C may be enough to prevent scurvy, but not enough to prevent fat oxidation. The results of oxidation may not show up for a long time, in the form of cancer or another debilitating disease—and then it may be too late.

Nutrition also plays an important role in the balance of fats in our body. Our blood contains a variety of fats (lipids) and fat-like substances. Although our body requires a certain amount of fat to function well, an excess of some types of fats have been implicated in cardiovascular disease. These "bad" fats, which clog up your arteries, include *serum cholesterol, low-density lipoproteins (LDL),* and *triglycerides. High-density lipoproteins (HDL)* are thought to be the "good" kind of cholesterol because they are associated with a lowered risk of heart disease. The balance between good and bad cholesterol is determined by several factors including diet, exercise, and heredity. We can manipulate two out of three of these factors to create a more desirable balance. For example, there is evidence that cholesterol and triglycerides can be lowered by certain supplements. These supplements, which include niacin, vitamins C and E, and chromium, may also lower LDL and raise HDL cholesterol. Aerobic exercise and a low-fat, high-fiber diet have also been shown to be effective. Simply reducing the amount of cholesterol in your diet is a rather ineffective way of changing your blood cholesterol levels. The most effective plan for lowering blood cholesterol includes *all* these measures.

The drugs used to lower cholesterol have some severe side effects, including gall bladder disease. Nutritional supplements have no severe side effects. This is why *The Journal of the American Medical Association* and *Postgraduate Medicine,* two highly respected professional journals, have published research papers that conclude that niacin is the treatment of choice for lowering blood serum cholesterol and triglycerides.

THE ODAs—
A REDEFINITION OF HEALTH

We have gradually expanded our knowledge and our thinking to include the notion that health should no longer be negatively defined as the absence of disease. Our current concept of real health is not one of mere survival—it is a positive state of total mental and physical well-being. We have drawn a distinction between maintaining *minimal* health—which is what the RDAs appear to do—and attaining and maintaining *optimal* health—which the RDAs do not necessarily ensure. We want to be as healthy as we can be in our daily lives. This includes taking advantage of the most current research on the prevention of disease and the integration of nutritional therapies with appropriate medical care during the early, most treatable stage of disease.

In order to attain this state of optimal health and disease prevention, we must take into our bodies *optimum*—not minimum—amounts of vitamins and minerals. To distinguish them from the lesser amounts characteristic of the RDAs, I have called these amounts the *Optimum Daily Allowances, or ODAs.* The need for ODAs is based on three factors: (1) We are not meeting the RDAs even if we are eating the "perfect" diet; (2) The foods available to us do not contain the amounts of vitamins and minerals they should contain because of many factors including loss of nutrients through shipping, storage, and processing; (3) We require higher levels of vitamins and minerals owing to the constant bombardment of stress factors in our environment such as pollution and emotional stress; and (4) Vitamins and minerals are never 100 percent absorbed.

The ODAs in this book are given as a range of dosages, in acknowledgment of the fact that people are individuals and so will require differing amounts. Although a few ODAs are close to or the same as the RDAs, they are generally in excess of the RDAs, often many times this amount. However, they are not "megadoses." Not only is this term too limiting—it is totally inaccurate. "Mega" has come to mean "ten times" in popular usage; however, it literally means "million." In *Design Your Own Vitamin and Mineral Program,* the ODA is often much higher than ten times the RDA; however, you will never be taking a million times the RDA of anything.

The ODAs are based on data from three sources: the most up-to-date research studies published in highly respected American and foreign professional journals; my own clinical experience; and the experiences of other well-known clinicians in the field. It has been estimated that our knowledge in the biological sciences is doubling every five to ten years, and human nutrition is an especially fast-growing field. I and other progressive practitioners are interested in new findings and new ideas. We prefer to look forward, rather than backward. This means that at this point in time, we are sometimes in the position of having to take sketchy, somewhat experimental data and applying them to real-life situations, perhaps before they are completely understood. So in many instances, I have had to take the research studies a step further.

One example of this is with the uses of vitamin C. It has been shown that vitamin C blocks nitrosamine formation from the nitrates in food, so it stands to reason that the same would hold true for nitrosamines formed from air pollution in our lungs. Another example is relying on animal studies. Wherever possible, human studies are used. However, sometimes animal studies are all we have to go on, in part because it would be unethical to use similar methods on humans. For instance, tumors are often induced in animals and then vitamins are given to assess their efficacy in suppressing tumor growth. The animals are usually killed after the experiment is completed to measure the effects of nutrition on various parts of the body. The practice of extrapolating information from animal studies and applying it to humans is firmly rooted in medicine. Most major breakthroughs in medicine have occurred as a consequence of animal research. The efficacy and toxicity of almost all the drugs used in medical practice were originally based on animal research. Animal studies have also been generally accepted as sufficient proof that certain substances may be cancer-producing in humans, such as cyclamates and red dye number 2. It is logical to conclude that in many cases extrapolation of data from animal studies with respect to human nutrition is just as valid.

Another type of study that the ODAs are based upon is the epidemiological study. An example of this is when researchers measure the level of a certain vitamin in the diet or blood of groups of people. They then see whether there is any correlation between these levels and their state of health. Many of the studies linking a higher level of vitamin A with a lower risk of cancer are of this type. In cases such as this, the RDAs and the ODAs may agree as to the usefulness of a vitamin or mineral, but not as to the amount.

Absorption is never 100 percent. For instance, only 60 percent of vitamin A is absorbed. In addition, individual requirements vary. Nobel Prize laureate Linus Pauling has recently shown that the vitamin requirements of individual animals within the same species vary by as much as 2000 percent. He extrapolates that the same is probably true for humans.

Nutritionists and physicians have disputed many of the findings of the epidemiologists and have demanded experimental "proof." D. M. Hegsted, writing in the Harvard School of Public Health's December 1985 issue of *Nutrition Reviews*, addressed this issue, pointing out the inconsistency in their reasoning. He notes that "there is a large body of science, as valid as any other science, which rests upon observation and deduction rather than experimentation—such as astronomy, geology, and archeology. Indeed, the crowning achievement of biology—the theory of evolution—is based upon observation and deduction."

Finally, while it is not a rule that more is always better, some experiments have shown that excesses of the RDA do have a greater positive effect than lower amounts. It is not true that taking supplements is a waste of time and money because you simply excrete the excess in your urine. Vitamins and minerals are generally excreted this way after your enzymes have been saturated and have realized the maximum potential of their specific uses. These range from stimulating your immune system to putting minerals in your bones. The beneficial effect of an excess of certain nutrients on the immune system has in fact been demonstrated. An example is vitamin C: Studies in which animals or humans were given substantially higher doses of the RDA for vitamin C have suggested that this excess, which spills into the urine, is not "wasted." Rather, it may have a protective effect against urinary and bladder cancer.

Our bodies have the remarkable ability to adapt and protect us from the ever-increasing abuses of life. Some people can tolerate a good deal of these insults while others are much more sensitive and need optimal nutritional protection. However, we have no way of knowing for sure who falls into which category. Taking the Optimum Daily Allowances given in this book means you are joining the legions of nutritionally aware people who would rather be safe than sorry.

Note: If you have any medical condition, please consult with your physician before taking any vitamin or mineral supplements. If he or she is not versed in nutrition, bring this book to the office. The ODAs are not meant to be a substitute for any medications, therapies, or any medical treatment. In most cases, they may be used in addition to the recommended medical treatment. However, once again, consult your physician first.

Chapter 4

HOW TO DESIGN
YOUR OWN
VITAMIN AND MINERAL
PROGRAM

You will find it easy to use this book to design your own vitamin and mineral program. To begin, I recommend that you first read through *Part Two: The Vitamins* and *Part Three: The Minerals* to get an overall picture of what vitamins and minerals can do for you. Then tear out the worksheet on pages 170–71 in *Part Four* and go through the book again, chapter by chapter, with pen or pencil in hand, filling in your individual Optimum Daily Allowance for each vitamin and mineral.

Remember: Never take just one vitamin or mineral, or just a select few. Although each has its own biochemical function in the body, nutrients tend to work together synergistically. They help each other. You must take appropriate amounts of them all, and in proportion to each other, to get the most out of them. In addition, because they compete for absorption in the body, supplementation of a single nutrient may put you at risk for developing an imbalance in those nutrients which are not being supplemented.

STEP 1: DETERMINE YOUR BASIC ODA. Notice that in each nutrient chapter, I first give a basic Optimum Daily Allowance. This is a safe dose range for general optimum health, and will help prevent illnesses in many people. Using the basic ODA program given in the sample worksheet on pages 170–71 as a guide, your first step is to fill in your basic ODA for each nutrient. If you are in good health, with no particular health concerns, and are primarily interested in all-round disease prevention, I advise you to start at the lower end of this basic ODA range. If you continue to feel well, this is probably all you need to take. If you are generally not feeling that well, I recommend you start at the low end and gradually increase the dosages until you notice an improvement in the way you feel. Space is provided on the blank worksheet for you to record your progress.

STEP 2: INDIVIDUALIZE YOUR ODA. Some people are at higher risk owing to personal or family health history, environmental pollution, or other forms of stress. That is why in each chapter I also give specific examples of amounts that I have found useful for preventing specific conditions and concerns. These ODAs for specific uses generally go higher than the basic ODAs because, in my experience, certain circumstances require higher amounts. Although they are higher than the ODAs, they are still nontoxic, with no adverse effects. In some cases, these higher amounts have also been effective as the primary treatment for an already existing condition, or are valuable as an adjunct to appropriate medical treatment.

However, large doses of certain vitamins or minerals may have undesirable effects in some individuals with medical conditions, or affect their medication. I cannot emphasize too strongly that if you have a suspected or diagnosed condition, it is for your own protection to see a qualified health practitioner for treatment. In general, pregnant women may safely take the low end of the basic ODA, but again, please check with your physician. For an example of the ODA program that would suit most pregnant women, see page 37.

So if you are at high risk for a particular disease, your next step is to decide how much more than the basic ODA you want to take of specific nutrients. For example, if cancer runs in your family, I recommend you take higher amounts of vitamins A, C, and E as well as the minerals zinc and selenium, because they have been shown to be protective against cancer. If you smoke, or live or work with a smoker, or live in a big city with polluted air, you also might want to take higher amounts of certain nutrients. The same goes for high blood pressure or other forms of coronary disease, diabetes, premenstrual syndrome, fibrocystic breast disease, and so on. To serve as a guide, I have provided special ODA programs for the most common specific concerns such as emotional stress, enhancing immunity, cancer prevention, cardiovascular disease prevention, skin problems, and diabetes prevention.

In addition, you can use the examples given below to get an idea of how supplement programs (along with a good diet and exercise program, of course) can be individualized for people in a variety of life circumstances.

I'll start with myself: I live and run my practice in New York City. I am under a lot of stress from my polluted environment and business pressures. I play tennis, lift weights, and get regular aerobic exercise. My diet is optimal (low fat, low sugar, high fiber), but there is a strong family propensity toward heart disease, high cholesterol, and high triglycerides. My supplement program looks like this:

vitamin A	5000 IU
beta-carotene	50,000 IU
B complex	50 mg
vitamin C	3000 mg (plus 1500 mg bioflavonoids)
vitamin D	400 IU
vitamin E	400 IU
calcium	1200 mg
magnesium	600 mg
phosphorus	(from diet)
zinc	50 mg
iron	25 mg
copper	(from diet)
manganese	25 mg
GTF chromium	400 mcg
selenium	200 mcg
iodine	150 mcg

My coauthor is in her thirties and is a professional in business for herself. She lives and works in New York City, and so is under stress similar to mine. She has been successfully treated with surgery and chemotherapy for breast cancer, and wants to keep it that way. She tends toward hormonal problems, premenstrual syndrome in particular. She eats an optimum diet, and gets regular aerobic exercise. Her program is:

vitamin A	10,000 IU
beta-carotene	75,000 IU
B complex	50 mg (plus 100 mg B-6)

vitamin C	5000–10,000 mg (to bowel tolerance) (plus 5000 mg bioflavonoids)
vitamin D	400 IU
vitamin E	1200 IU
calcium	1200 mg
magnesium	600 mg
phosphorus	(from diet)
zinc	50 mg
iron	25 mg
copper	(from diet)
manganese	30 mg
GTF chromium	200 mcg
selenium	400 mcg
iodine	150 mcg

R.M. is a twenty-five-year-old woman who lives and works as a secretary in the suburbs. She gets very little exercise and is overweight. She has no health complaints and does not feel particularly stressed about anything other than her weight and her craving for sweets. Her program is:

vitamin A	5000 IU
beta-carotene	10,000 IU
B complex	25 mg
vitamin C	1000 mg (plus 500 mg bioflavonoids)
vitamin D	400 IU
vitamin E	400 IU
calcium	1000 mg
magnesium	500 mg
phosphorus	(from diet)
zinc	22.5 mg
iron	25 mg
copper	2 mg
manganese	15 mg
GTF chromium	600 mcg

selenium	100 mcg
iodine	300 mcg

J.S. is a thirty-five-year-old businessman who lives and works in Los Angeles. His brother and father have a history of bowel cancer, and he is quite worried that he will get it too, especially since he has a history of spastic colitis. He does not eat an optimal diet or get regular exercise; however, he is willing to make changes. His program is:

vitamin A	10,000 IU
beta-carotene	50,000 IU
B complex	50 mg
vitamin C	5000 mg (plus 2500 mg bioflavonoids)
vitamin D	400 IU
vitamin E	800 IU
calcium	1000 mg
magnesium	500 mg
phosphorus	(from diet)
zinc	50 mg
iron	15 mg
copper	2 mg
manganese	15 mg
GTF chromium	200 mcg
selenium	300 mcg
iodine	50 mcg

S.S. is a sixty-seven-year-old retired teacher with osteoporosis and arthritis. She has become interested in nutrition over the years and eats a good diet, but she cannot eat more than 1200 calories a day because she is sedentary and is worried about gaining weight. She refuses to take drugs. Her program is:

vitamin A	10,000 IU
beta-carotene	10,000 IU
B complex	100 mg

vitamin C . . . .   5000 mg (plus 5000 mg bioflavonoids)
vitamin D . . . .   800 IU
vitamin E . . . .   1200 IU
calcium . . . .   2000 mg
magnesium . . . .   1000 mg
phosphorus . . . .   400 mg
zinc . . . .   50 mg
iron . . . .   25 mg
copper . . . .   2 mg
manganese . . . .   30 mg
GTF chromium . . . . . .   200 mcg
selenium . . . .   200 mcg
iodine . . . .   300 mcg

E.B. is a sixteen-year-old high school student. In addition to his school work, he has daily practice and training for the basketball team. He is very stressed, always feels in a rush, and often feels tired. His physician has diagnosed iron-deficiency anemia; he feels he is underweight. E.B. skips breakfast and eats school lunches. Dinner is the only good meal he eats, since his mother cooks it. His program is:

vitamin A . . . .   5000 IU
beta-carotene . . . .   10,000 IU
B complex . . . .   50 mg
vitamin C . . . .   3000 mg
vitamin D . . . .   400 IU
vitamin E . . . .   400 IU
calcium . . . .   1500 mg
magnesium . . . .   750 mg
phosphorus . . . .   400 mg
zinc . . . .   30 mg
iron . . . .   30 mg
copper . . . .   2 mg
manganese . . . .   15 mg

GTF chromium . . . . . . 400 mcg

selenium . . . . 100 mcg

iodine . . . . 50 mcg

J.Y. is twenty-seven years old and pregnant. She has quit her job and has plenty of time to cook and plan her meals, but she is concerned about excessive weight gain. She doesn't want to eat over 1800 calories a day nor drink more than two cups of low-fat milk. Her program is:

vitamin A . . . . 5000 IU

beta-carotene . . . . 5000 IU

B complex . . . . 25 mg (plus 800 mcg folic acid)

vitamin C . . . . 1000 mg (plus 500 mg bioflavonoids)

vitamin D . . . . 200 IU

vitamin E . . . . 400 IU

calcium . . . . 1000 mg

magnesium . . . . 500 mg

phosphorus . . . . (from diet)

zinc . . . . 22.5 mg

iron . . . . 30 mg

copper . . . . 2 mg

manganese . . . . 15 mg

GTF chromium . . . . . . 200 mcg

selenium . . . . 100 mcg

iodine . . . . 150 mcg

M.R. is a thirty-eight-year-old underweight man who lives and works in Chicago. His job as a postal worker means he has irregular hours which have affected his eating habits. He worries about his blood pressure, which is slightly elevated. I would recommend the following program for him:

vitamin A . . . . 5000 IU

beta-carotene . . . . 25,000 IU

B complex . . . . 200 mg

vitamin C . . . . 3000 mg (plus 1500 mg bioflavonoids) vitamin D . . . .   400 IU

vitamin E . . . .   400 IU

calcium . . . .   1500 mg

magnesium . . . .   750 mg

phosphorus . . . .   (from diet)

zinc . . . .   22.5 mg

iron . . . .   15 mg

copper . . . .   2 mg

manganese . . . .   15 mg

GTF chromium . . . . . .   200 mcg

selenium . . . .   100 mcg

iodine . . . .   150 mcg

potassium . . . .   from potassium-rich foods; also reduce
sodium in diet

J.K. is seventeen years old and living away from home at a college in the country. Her diet is poor and she must rely mostly on cafeteria food. Since beginning to take birth control pills, she has noticed some water retention, mild depression, and cramps during menstruation.

vitamin A . . . .   5000 IU

beta-carotene . . . .   10,000 IU

B complex . . . .   100 mg

vitamin C . . . .   3000 mg (plus 1500 mg bioflavonoids)

vitamin D . . . .   400 IU

vitamin E . . . .   400 IU

calcium . . . .   1500 mg

magnesium . . . .   750 mg

phosphorus . . . .   (from diet)

zinc . . . .   50 mg

iron . . . .   25 mg

copper . . . .   (from diet)

manganese . . . .   30 mg

GTF chromium . . . . . .   400 mcg

selenium . . . . 200 mcg

iodine . . . . 150 mcg

R.S. lives in the suburbs. He has become sedentary since his recent retirement from the police force and is feeling depressed. He complains of joint and lower-back pain. He smokes cigarettes. His program is:

vitamin A . . . . 10,000 IU

beta-carotene . . . . 50,000 IU

B complex . . . . 150 mg

vitamin C . . . . 3000 mg (plus 1500 mg bioflavonoids)

vitamin D . . . . 400 IU

vitamin E . . . . 800 IU

calcium . . . . 1200 mg

magnesium . . . . 600 mg

phosphorus . . . . (from diet)

zinc . . . . 50 mg

iron . . . . 15 mg

copper . . . . 2 mg

manganese . . . . 30 mg

GTF chromium . . . . . . 200 mcg

selenium . . . . 300 mcg

iodine . . . . 150 mcg

STEP 3: MATCH YOUR ODAs WITH YOUR SUPPLE-MENTS. The simplest, easiest way to obtain your own ODA is by starting with a good multivitamin formula which combines a number of nutrients in one tablet. Generally, the multivitamin preparations currently available are your basic source of B-complex, vitamin A, D, and E. Some may contain enough vitamin C for some people. They may also include negligible amounts of minerals—less than the RDA, although they might contain the RDAs of iron and zinc. Therefore, I also advise my patients to buy a good multimineral tablet in addition to their multivitamin tablet.

Look for multivitamin and multimineral preparations with labeling that implies high potency, for example, "extra potency," "megavitamins," or "therapeutic formula." Together they will take care of most of the nutrients covered in this book. Depending upon their potency and your Optimum Daily Amount as specified in your program, you may need to take one, two, or more a day of such a formula in order to get the basic amount of each nutrient that is right for you. Unfortunately, it is impossible to design a single pill that contains optimum amounts of everything you need while keeping it small enough to swallow.

Having settled on a basic formula, you can then further customize your program by adding to the general supplement those individual nutrients you feel you need more of. For example, your multivitamin may contain 25,000 IU of vitamin A. If you want to take a total of 50,000 IU because you have acne, you can add 25,000 IU of vitamin A. If your general supplement has 200 micrograms of chromium and you have diabetes, you might want to add 400 micrograms of chromium for a total of 600 micrograms per day.

WORKING WITH YOUR
HEALTH CARE PRACTITIONER

If you prefer to work with a nutritionist, it is very important that you ask about his or her background. A qualified nutritionist may have a bachelor's degree, a master's degree, or a doctorate in nutrition from an accredited school. In addition, if their educational experience has met the guidelines of the American Dietetic Association, they may qualify to take the registered dietitian (R.D.) exam, which assures a certain level of educational and occupational experience.

Unfortunately, most physicians are not well versed in nutrition. Although this is lamentable, it is completely understandable and is in large part due to inadequate nutritional education in medical school. Nutrition is generally offered as an elective to medical students, and the entire course usually consists of a grand total of three hours. Also, medical training emphasizes the diagnosis and treatment of disease, rather than its prevention.

The ideal situation is to have your physician working with your nutritionist, particularly if you have a medical condition. This is the situation with many of my patients, and it can work out beautifully. You can't expect your physician to know and do everything. When we read medical literature, we tend to read what is most relevant to our specialty. Even though much of the research in this book is from widely read and respected medical journals, your physician may not be familiar with the studies. For example, when I read *The Journal of the American Medical Association,* I naturally read the research pertaining to nutrition, rather than the latest surgical developments. There simply isn't the time to read all the research about every specialty. However, it *is* reasonable to expect your physician to be open-minded about the nutritional approach, since nutritional research is widespread throughout the medical literature.

HOW AND WHEN TO TAKE SUPPLEMENTS

Your body can absorb and use only so much of a vitamin or mineral at one time. So to increase the utilization of these nutrients, try to divide the dosage over the course of the day, especially if you are working with the higher doses. For example, if you are taking a total of 3000 milligrams of vitamin C daily, take 1000 milligrams three times a day. In addition, supplements are best taken at mealtime, along with your food. This increases absorption and prevents the indigestion that sometimes occurs when supplements are taken on an empty stomach. You may take your supplements a few minutes before a meal, or up to a half hour after a meal.

There has been a lot of confusing information published about the interference of certain nutrients with the absorption of others. In my opinion, the evidence is not strong enough for me to advise not taking certain vitamins and minerals together, or with certain foods. As I say to my patients, nature supplies us with a variety of nutrients in each meal, so why should taking supplements together pose a realistic problem? Life is complicated enough without your having to worry about whether your bran muffin is interfering with your absorption of calcium.

HOW DO YOU KNOW WHETHER
YOUR SUPPLEMENTS ARE WORKING?

People who are taking supplements for general good health and disease prevention usually just feel better. They feel calmer, get fewer colds, have more energy, and have a general sense of well-being. Even my patients who were resistant to taking supplements have confessed this to me. These people sometimes go off their vitamins and minerals for a while, and then come back to me and say, "You know, skeptical as I was, I must admit the supplements did make a difference in the way I felt." Because of our naturally longer life spans, there are no long-term studies that show that vitamin supplementation actually increases longevity. However, some studies show that diet and vitamin intake influences the life span of animals. In one experiment, mice that were given four times the RDA of vitamins lived almost 20 percent longer than those given the RDA.

If you are taking supplements to prevent a specific condition, and the condition fails to materialize, there is, of course, no way of knowing for sure whether the supplements "worked" or whether you would have remained healthy anyway. For people who take vitamins and minerals as a kind of "health insurance," no news is good news.

In other cases, when you are taking supplements for a specific condition, you will know whether they are working because you will have tangible confirmation—your condition will improve. If you have a skin problem, and you take extra vitamin A, it is working if your skin clears up; if you have high blood pressure and you take extra calcium, magnesium, and vitamin D (and hopefully modify your diet) and your blood pressure improves, these nutrients are obviously working in your favor.

Vitamins and minerals do not work overnight! If you are nervous and irritable today and take a B complex tonight, do not expect to feel calm and serene tomorrow. You must give them time—but do not wait forever. In general, three or four weeks is enough time for you to see beneficial effects from a supplement. One exception is with premenstrual syndrome. You need at least two menstrual cycles to determine if B-complex supplementation is effective.

If you begin at the lower end of the ODA range and you see no results at this dose, you may escalate the dosage and give it another few weeks. Keep raising the dosage, if necessary, until you reach the highest range of the ODA. Give that another month or so, unless you start noticing some adverse effects. For example, if you are taking beta-carotene for acne, you might start at 50,000 IU per day. If after a couple of weeks you see some improvement, but nothing spectacular, you may try going up to 75,000 IU for a while. If your skin clears up more, you might want to go up to 100,000 IU to see if that will improve it even further. If your skin begins to look slightly yellow or orange (the only adverse effect of beta-carotene), you should then cut back to 75,000 IU. If you have gone up to the maximum safe dosage and have stayed there for a month or two, but have seen no results, I would suggest you cut back gradually to a more moderate level. Obviously, large doses do not work in your case and you should try some other means of controlling your condition.

Vitamin and mineral supplementation is an ongoing, evolving process. Your body changes with time, and your need for supplements may too. You might, for instance, want to increase your Optimum Daily Allowance of B complex and/or vitamin C during times of illness or extreme stress. Take a look at how you feel; see whether whatever you are working on has improved. Obviously, you want to take the smallest amount needed to improve a particular condition. Why take 75,000 IU of vitamin A if 50,000 or 25,000 work fine? Generally, one can take a supplement for a specific problem for six months. After that, try lowering the dosage. If the condition returns, return to the higher dosage—that's your body telling you that's how much you need.

ARE VITAMINS AND MINERALS HARMFUL?

Some people are afraid that they will overdose on vitamins and minerals and cause their bodies some harm. Such caveats fall especially from the lips of nutritionally unsophisticated practitioners; they are then passed on to the public by the media. The facts are that only a few vitamins and minerals have *any* known toxicities, all of which are reversible, with the exception of vitamin D.

Anything can be harmful if you take enough of it—even pure water! But vitamins and minerals are among the safest substances on earth. The amounts needed to become toxic are enormous. There are no studies that indicate that the ODAs in this book would create any toxicity in a normal adult. By "normal" I mean that you are not on any medication, and do not have a medical condition. These factors can influence your vitamin and mineral requirements by making them higher or lower. I have included some data about these requirements; however you should consult your physician for specifics if you have any questions.

You may be concerned that it is possible for your body to grow dependent on large amounts of vitamins or minerals after a while. There is very little convincing evidence of this. There is some indication that certain individuals who take very high doses of vitamin C and then suddenly stop run the risk of having symptoms of rebound scurvy. This is not well proven. However, common sense dictates that it is not wise to stop anything "cold turkey" if you have been taking it into your body for a prolonged period of time. This holds true for drugs—Valium, hormones such as cortisone, and many psychiatric drugs—and for switching your car from high-octane to low-octane fuel. Why should it be any different with vitamins? If your body has been finely tuned and is accustomed to having an optimal amount of a certain nutrient, it naturally must adjust when you change the way you are feeding it.

Therefore, if you want to cut back for any reason, it is logical to "wean" yourself away from supplements gradually. I generally recommended stepping down every two weeks until you reach your desired new level. For instance, many people increase their intake of vitamin C during the cold and flu season. If you have been taking 5000 milligrams of vitamin C every day during the winter, you may cut down to 4000 milligrams for two weeks, then to 3000 milligrams for the next two weeks, then 2000 milligrams, and so on.

If you're traveling and want to reduce your dosages because of the inconvenience, it is generally safe to cut your doses in half during this time. Nothing dramatic will happen if you forget to take your vitamins for a day every once in a while, either. Even the water-soluble vitamins remain in the body for two days or so, so you do have a margin of safety.

A GUIDE TO BUYING SUPPLEMENTS

One of the most common questions my patients ask me is: "Should I buy 'natural' or 'synthetic' vitamins?" As far as we know, there doesn't seem to be much difference between a vitamin found in food and one that is made in the laboratory. They are essentially the same chemical, made of the same molecules. The fat-soluble vitamins may be the exception: There is some evidence that the naturally occurring form of vitamin E is more absorbable and biologically active.

However, the word "natural" on the label does *not* necessarily mean that all the vitamin in the bottle is simply extracted from a natural food source. In fact, most so-called natural vitamins actually contain a large amount of synthetic vitamins. The reasons for this are primarily economic: If vitamin C supplements, for example, were derived solely from rose hips, the cost would be enormous.

The term "natural" really refers to the fact that the supplement does not contain other unnatural ingredients. Here there is a difference: Supplements that are not labeled "natural" may also include coal tars, artificial coloring, preservatives, sugars, starch, and sometimes other additives.

This is why I generally recommend "natural" vitamins. Why take these potentially harmful substances into the body when you don't have to?

Mineral supplements may be chelated, meaning surrounded by a carrier protein which transports the mineral to the bloodstream, in an attempt to enhance absorption. This process also increases their price. Unfortunately, studies on the absorbability of the various forms of mineral supplements are rather sparse at this time. I cannot recommend chelated minerals across the board; however, some combinations have been shown to be more absorbable. Unfortunately, they are often more expensive and may not be cost effective. If the difference in price is not enormous, you may prefer to buy chelated minerals for possible enhanced absorption. Keep in mind that if you take supplements with a meal, they are usually automatically chelated in your stomach during digestion.

Some supplements are available in a time-release formula in an attempt to release the nutrients gradually. This sounds fine in theory; however in practice it may actually decrease absorption and so I do not recommend time-release over regular formulas. Studies have shown that time-released vitamin C did not raise blood levels of vitamin C as effectively as non-time-released supplements. In another study, time-released niacin had less of a beneficial effect on blood cholesterols than non-time-released.

HOW LONG DO SUPPLEMENTS LAST?

Vitamins and minerals do not last forever; their potency gradually diminishes over a period of time. Vitamins, unopened, generally last for about two years; opened, they generally last for about one year. Mineral supplements last longer, and usually it is not the minerals themselves that go bad —it is the other substances in the supplement, such as the chelating agents, which spoil.

Vitamin and mineral supplements should be stored in a cool, dry, dark place. The refrigerator usually has a lot of moisture in it, and is quite cold, which could affect certain vitamins, so I don't recommend this as a storage place. Many people keep their supplements on top of the refrigerator; however, this location is generally too warm. A room temperature closet is usually fine.

Many people transfer their supplements to smaller, more convenient containers for work and travel. If the container is opaque and closes tightly, supplements can be stored in them for several months without losing much of their potency.

Chapter 5

YOUR TOTAL
HEALTH PLAN

Taking supplements is not a carte blanche for you to eat and drink anything you want; nor is it a panacea for all your ills. Vitamins and mineral
supplements are just that—*supplements*. They work best when they are a
part of a well-rounded plan for optimum health. Along with your supplements, it is important for you also to eat wholesome foods, get a reasonable amount of exercise, and maintain a healthy, wholesome lifestyle that
includes no smoking, a minimum of alcohol and other drugs, and stress
management.

THE BASIC INTELLIGENT DIET

For all their value, vitamin and mineral supplements do not take the place
of good fresh food. In the first place, you still need a balanced amount of
carbohydrates, fats, and proteins. In the second place, by eating nutritious
foods you are assured of at least getting some vitamins and minerals in
their natural form. This is important because when these nutrients are
ingested as part of the food in which they are naturally found, they are
generally absorbed and utilized better. In addition, by taking supplements
along with nutritious foods, you will enhance the absorption of the nutrients the supplements contain as well. Taking supplements after eating a
bowl of low-fat yogurt mixed with fresh fruit would probably result in
more of the nutrients being absorbed than if you took them with a couple
of commercially prepared cookies or a bag of potato chips.

Finally, there is so much we still don't know about food. There are
bound to be substances that have as yet been undiscovered—and if we
don't know about them, how can you possibly expect to get them from a
pill? These factors may have many important effects on the body. For
example, recently studies have shown there is a connection between a high

intake of cruciferous vegetables (these include cabbage, broccoli, cauli-flower) and a lowered risk of several types of cancer. This is an example of an important health effect that cannot be totally explained on the basis of our present knowledge of nutrients.

What follows is the "Basic Intelligent Diet" I recommend for most of my patients, in addition to their Optimum Daily Allowance of vitamins and minerals. It is basically a high-fiber, low-fat, low-sugar eating plan that is moderate in protein.

A Few Basic Rules to Remember

1) Avoid processed foods such as white flour, sugar, and processed cheese. Use whole grain rice, breads, and cereals.

2) Use whole fresh foods rather than canned, frozen, or commercially prepared foods.

3) Minimize salt. Foods naturally contain some salt, so try not to add any extra. Substitute salt-free spices and herbs such as garlic, pepper, and lemon juice.

4) Avoid sugar. You may substitute honey, maple syrup, or blackstrap molasses, but use these sparingly. Many people consume too much fruit, and consequently too much sugar. One glass of natural, unsweetened juice contains the equivalent of three to four fruits! Try mixing juice with club soda or water so it is not as sweet and concentrated.

5) Cook food quickly, using a minimum of fat or water to preserve as many nutrients as possible. Eat vegetables raw or steamed. Foods may also be baked, or quickly stir-fried in a small amount of oil.

6) Use butter and oils sparingly. Do not use margarine, which contains oil that has been hydrogenated.

7) Minimize high-fat meats such as pork, lamb, and beef.

8) Eat slowly. Enjoy your food! The slower you eat, the less you eat.

9) Minimize coffee, tea, sodas, other caffeine- and sugar-containing bever-ages, and chocolate. Natural fruit juice (up to one cup per day), club soda or seltzer, herbal teas, grain-type coffee substitute, and filtered or bottled water are preferable.

DAILY MENUS

WOMEN: These amounts are for women 5 feet 3 inches to 5 feet 9 inches. If you are over 5 feet 9 inches, add one portion each of vegetable and fiber. If you are under 5 feet 3 inches, subtract one portion each of vegetable and fiber.

8 ounces of low-fat milk or yogurt, or 1/2 cup low-fat cottage cheese

3 cups of nonstarchy vegetables: lettuce, zucchini, tomato, broccoli, cucumber, cabbage, etc.

2 fresh fruits

4–5 fiber servings*

2–3 ounces of protein food at each meal (seafood, fish, eggs, nonprocessed low-fat cheese, yogurt, milk, tofu, chicken, turkey)

MEN: These amounts are for men 5 feet 10 inches to 6 feet and up. If you are under 5 feet 10 inches, subtract one serving each of vegetable and fiber.

8 ounces of low-fat milk or yogurt, or 1/2 cup cottage cheese

5 cups of nonstarchy vegetables

3–4 fresh fruits

7–8 fiber servings*

3–4 ounces protein at each meal

* The following are equivalent to one fiber serving:

1/2 cup pasta, rice, or other grain

1 slice bread

1 small potato or ear of corn

1/2 cup granola (low-sugar)

1/2 cup winter squash

1/4 cup yam or sweet potato

1/2 cup peas, beans, or lentils

1 cup puffed cereal

1 1/2 tablespoons nut butter, or 20 nuts (no oil added; no more than one
    serving per day)

SAMPLE MENU 1

WOMEN: 1200 calories   **MEN**: 1800 calories

Breakfast:

2 slices whole wheat bread   3 slices whole wheat bread
3 ounces Jarlsberg cheese   4 ounces Jarlsberg cheese
2 slices tomato   3 slices tomato

Lunch:

1 cup fresh salad or vegetables   2 cups salad or vegetables
3 ounces baked fish   4 ounces baked fish
1 medium baked potato   1 medium baked potato

Dinner:

3 ounces broiled chicken   4 ounces broiled chicken
2 cups salad or vegetables   2 cups salad or vegetables
1 cup brown rice   2 cups brown rice

Snacks:

1/2 cup low-fat cottage cheese   1 cup low-fat cottage cheese
1 medium pear   1 medium pear
1 teaspoon oat bran or wheat   1 tablespoon oat bran or wheat
    germ   germ

SAMPLE MENU 2

WOMEN: 1200 calories   **MEN: 1800 calories**

Breakfast:

1 cup puffed rice cereal   1 1/2 cups puffed rice cereal
1/2 banana   1 banana
1/2 cup low-fat milk or yogurt   1 cup low-fat milk or yogurt

Lunch:

1 cup fresh salad or vegetables   1 cup lentil soup
3 ounces chicken on 2 slices   4 ounces chicken on 2 slices
  whole wheat bread   whole wheat bread
                                    2 cups salad or vegetables

Dinner:

1 cup pasta with tomato sauce   2 cups pasta with tomato sauce
3 ounces broiled filet of sole   4 ounces broiled filet of sole
2 cups salad or vegetables   2 cups salad or vegetables

Snacks:

1/2 cup low-fat yogurt   1 cup low-fat yogurt
1 medium apple   1 medium apple
1 teaspoon oat bran   1 tablespoon oat bran

Note: If butter, oil, or dressings are used, add 100 calories per serving. You may also have an additional 1/2 cup of fruit juice diluted with water or club soda.

There is good evidence that 70 to 80 percent of all cancers are produced by diet, nutrition, lifestyle, and chemicals and other events in our environment. According to the National Academy of Sciences, up to 60 percent of cancer is due to nutritional factors alone. In a commentary in the *American Journal of Clinical Nutrition*, the author says, "Considering the overriding importance of the major chronic disease—coronary heart disease, hypertension, cancer, diabetes, and obesity—which will attack the great majority of Americans, nutrition-related activities are underfunded and only beginning to receive appropriate attention. Because of the prevalence of the chronic diseases, prevention must have a high priority. Nutrition offers one of the few, perhaps even the only, preventive avenues available."

While we wish there were better studies available in some cases, and surely they are forthcoming, there is clearly enough evidence to support the judicious use of vitamin and mineral supplements as part of a total health improvement program. The risks are negligible, but the possible benefits are great.

PART TWO
THE VITAMINS

FAT-SOLUBLE VITAMINS

Chapter 6

VITAMIN A

Many of the subclinical deficiency symptoms and health-building uses for vitamin A are related to the role it plays in our immune system and in the formation of healthy epithelial tissue. Epithelial tissue is found almost everywhere in the body—in the skin, the glands, the mucous membranes, the lining of the hollow organs, and along the entire length of the respiratory, gastrointestinal, and genitourinary tracts.

In many animal studies, vitamin A has been shown to improve resistance to infections and is especially useful in preventing both infectious and noninfectious diseases of the respiratory system. In my clinical experience I have found that vitamin A supplementation is an excellent and safe immune system booster. Patients who get frequent sore throats, colds, flu, sinusitis, or bronchitis have shown a marked decrease in the frequency and severity of these respiratory infections. I have also found that vitamin A supplementation is effective in decreasing the symptoms associated with allergic reactions, emphysema, and asthma. Chronic infections and illnesses can reduce the body's levels of vitamin A, thereby weakening the mucous membranes, making them more susceptible to viral infection.

There is also a growing interest in this vitamin as a cancer preventive, and there is enough evidence to suggest that it does offer protection from certain forms of this disease. For example, studies have shown that vitamin A lowers the incidence of lung cancer in men who smoke. But vitamin A may prove valuable for people who don't smoke, too. Air pollution contains toxic substances which are also found in cigarette smoke, such as tar and carbon monoxide. Therefore, I recommend vitamin A to my patients because it may also be useful for protecting against lung cancer due to air pollution. Vitamin A may also protect against the "secondhand" cigarette smoke that is inadvertently inhaled by nonsmokers. It has been shown that vitamin A is protective against gastrointestinal ulcers. Since people with ulcers are more prone to gastrointestinal cancer, this nutrient may also reduce the incidence of this type of cancer. Vitamin A appears to lower the incidence of breast cancer in women as well.

There may be other mechanisms at work in vitamin A's ability to work against the development and spread of cancer. It is an antioxidant, which protects our cells from the type of cell damage that leads to cancer. In animal studies it slowed the spread of breast cancer to other parts of the body. Interestingly, in a study of women with breast cancer undergoing chemotherapy, the women with higher blood levels of vitamin A responded twice as well to the drug treatment as did women with lower levels. There are two theories as to why these results were obtained: Vitamin A helped protect the women from the toxicity of the drugs, and/or the vitamin may have interacted with the drugs to increase their effectiveness. Nancy Bruning, who had chemotherapy for breast cancer before this study was published, luckily was taking vitamin A supplements during her therapy. I find it interesting that her side effects were relatively minor and she has no evidence of disease at this time, six years after her diagnosis.

Studies indicate that vitamin A is useful in promoting healthy cell growth, and is essential not only for healthy eyes but for healthy skin as well. It is therefore often used to treat acne. The type of vitamin A prescribed to treat severe forms of acne medically is a synthetic analog of vitamin A called *cis-retinoic acid*. This form is available only by prescription, and was developed so that the vitamin could be administered in very high doses—200,000 to 300,000 IU—without the level of toxicity that other active forms of vitamin A would bring about. Although this treatment is quite successful, there are still toxicity problems with this form. Beta-carotene, a "provitamin" or precursor of vitamin A from which your body makes active vitamin A, is nontoxic. When using beta-carotene, I have not needed to exceed 100,000 IU per day, and have gotten excellent results. I must point out that beta-carotene works even for patients with severe acne that has not improved significantly with medical treatment, including antibiotics. I have also found beta-carotene to be a useful, nontoxic treatment for dry skin, eczema, and psoriasis.

The traditionally recognized deficiency symptoms of vitamin A are night blindness and other eye problems, skin disorders, suboptimal growth, and reproductive failure. Low-level night blindness is becoming more common in the United States and may eventually become recognized as a subclinical deficiency. To prevent these severe deficiencies, the RDA is 5000 IU for men and 4000 IU for women (5000 for lactating women).

Food Sources: Active vitamin A is found only in animal sources. It is especially high in the fish liver oil from cod, halibut, salmon, and shark; it is also found in beef and chicken liver; and in eggs and dairy products. Beta-carotene, the vitamin A precursor, is found only in fruits and vegetables: green and yellow-orange vegetables and fruits such as carrots, kale, kohlrabi, parsley, spinach, turnip greens, dandelion greens, apricots, and cantaloupe.

When relying on food sources, be aware that vitamin A or beta-carotene can be destroyed by heat, alkali (such as baking soda added to cooking vegetables to keep them green), light, and air. Beta-carotene is especially susceptible to oxidation so carrot juice is rich in this substance only if it is fresh-pressed and you drink it immediately.

OPTIMUM DAILY ALLOWANCE—ODA

For optimum general health, the basic Optimum Daily Allowance for vitamin A (preferably at least half of which should be in the form of beta-carotene) is:

   10,000–50,000 IU for men and women

(It is recommended that pregnant and lactating women not exceed 10,000 IU per day, as vitamin A may cause birth defects or be toxic to the infant.)

In my clinical experience, I have found the following amounts of vitamin A to be valuable for:

Enhancing immunity . . . . 10,000–50,000 IU

Respiratory problems: (sinusitis, bronchitis,
   emphysema, allergies, asthma) . . . . 50,000–100,000 IU

Cancer prevention . . . . 50,000–100,000 IU

Gastrointestinal ulcers . . . . 50,000 IU

Skin problems: dry skin . . . . 25,000–50,000 IU

   acne, eczema, psoriasis . . . . 50,000–100,000 IU

Polluted air . . . . 10,000–25,000 IU

Remember: If you have a medical condition, please consult with your physician before taking supplements.

SUPPLEMENTS

Since active vitamin A (from fish liver oil) and beta-carotene may have slightly different functions in the body, I recommend that individuals get their total daily amount of vitamin A by taking a combination of both. For example, vitamin A studies that have been done with respect to cancer have correlated a high beta-carotene intake more often than fish liver oil vitamin A with a decreased risk of cancer. My own clinical experience is that beta-carotene taken with active vitamin A is the most effective way to supplement this vitamin. Palmitate, the synthetic form, is water miscible and is therefore preferable for people who have difficulty absorbing fats.

TOXICITY AND ADVERSE EFFECTS

Naturally occurring active vitamin A (from fish liver oil) is fat soluble and stored in the liver; it can, therefore, be toxic in large amounts. Palmitate, the synthetic form of active vitamin A, is also stored in the liver and so, like natural vitamin A, palmitate can be toxic.

Reports of 50,000 IU of active vitamin A causing toxicity are rare, except in infants, where 15,000 IU would cause problems. You must take at least 100,000 IU of *active* vitamin A daily for a period of months in order to display any signs of toxicity. Early signs of toxicity are fatigue, nausea, vomiting, headache, vertigo, blurred vision, muscular incoordination, and loss of body hair. All these symptoms are reversible when vitamin A supplementation is stopped.

Beta-carotene, on the other hand, can be given for long periods of time virtually without risk of toxicity. Since beta-carotene is a naturally occurring pigment, the only adverse effect of eating too much beta-carotene is the possibility of *carotenemia,* a harmless condition in which the skin turns a slight orange color. I often tell patients if they get carotenemia to cut back on their beta-carotene since this pigment indicates the body has converted as much beta-carotene to active A as it can. On the other hand, pigments such as carotenes are often given to sun-sensitive individuals since the tinting of the skin affords some additional protection against sunburn. Carotene preparations are also used by some people for a cosmetic effect: the slight tint looks like a suntan, and also allows them to tan more easily.

Chapter 7

VITAMIN D

Vitamin D is not truly a vitamin for two reasons: In its active form it is considered to be a hormone; and our bodies can make it from sunlight.

Vitamin D is primarily involved in the metabolism of calcium and phosphorus in the body. It increases the absorption of these minerals from the intestine and increases the uptake of minerals by the bones.

In children, rickets is the classical deficiency disease of this vitamin; the symptoms are stunted growth, delayed tooth development, weakness, softened skulls (in infants), and irreversible bone deformities. In adults, women with a history of vitamin D deficiency have difficulty giving birth because of irregularities in the pelvic bones.

In adults, *hypocalcemia* (low level of calcium in the bloodstream), *osteomalacia* (reduction in the mineral content of the bone), and *osteoporosis* (reduction in total bone mass) are associated with vitamin D deficiencies. Thinning bones, which fracture more easily, have recently been recognized as a growing problem in menopausal women. (Men can suffer, too, but women are more often affected because of the role that estrogen plays.) Calcium, magnesium, as well as other minerals and vitamins should be given along with vitamin D to treat these conditions, as they all work hand in hand in the body to form and maintain bone mass.

Recently, other studies have turned up possible additional roles that vitamin D plays. For example, vitamin D combined with calcium has been found to possess anticancer properties. In some people, low vitamin D has been linked with high blood pressure. Active vitamin D plays a role in the treatment of some immunological disorders. It may also improve muscle strength.

There is no RDA for vitamin D; however, the amount generally agreed upon by most professionals is 400 IU per day.

Food Sources: Food sources are generally low in this vitamin. The richest sources of vitamin D are fish liver oils and fatty saltwater fish such as sea bass, halibut, swordfish, herring, tuna, cod, and sable. Because milk is usually fortified with vitamin D, milk and dairy products are also a good source of this vitamin.

OPTIMUM DAILY ALLOWANCE—ODA

For optimum general health, the basic Optimum Daily Allowance for vitamin D is:

400–600 IU for men and women

In my clinical experience, I have found the following amounts of vitamin D to be valuable for:

Osteoporosis .... 400–600 IU
High blood pressure .... 400–600 IU

Remember: If you have a medical condition, please consult your physician before taking supplements.

Lifestyles, skin color, degree of air pollution, and geographical latitude all affect the degree of exposure to the sun, and therefore the amount of vitamin D we are able to make in our bodies. It is also questionable whether any vitamin D is synthesized during the winter months, and whether the body stores of this vitamin are able to meet the daily requirement during this period. Therefore, if you rarely go outdoors in the sunlight, have dark skin, live in the northern latitudes, avoid fortified dairy products, or have liver or kidney disease, you may be marginally deficient in this vitamin.

Recent research indicates that the elderly may be at high risk for vitamin D deficiency. Anyone with osteoporosis who has not responded to calcium supplementation may be advised to add moderate vitamin D supplementation, magnesium, and increased sunlight exposure to the regimen. One study suggested that elderly women may actually require 600–800 IU, rather than 400 IU per day. Most patients with Crohn's disease have deficient levels of vitamin D and should be supplemented with vitamin D to prevent osteomalacia.

SUPPLEMENTS

There are two forms of vitamin D. Vitamin D-3 is preferable since it is the naturally occurring form. Both D-3 and D-2, a synthetic form, become the active hormone vitamin D after passing through the liver and kidney. Special "active" forms are available by prescription for patients with chronic liver or kidney disease, because their ability to convert vitamin D may be impaired.

TOXICITY AND ADVERSE EFFECTS

According to several studies, up to 1000 IU per day of vitamin D appears to be safe. Both the beneficial and adverse effects of exceeding this amount are controversial. Overdosing of vitamin D is *irreversible and may be fatal.* Symptoms of too much vitamin D are nausea, loss of appetite, headache, diarrhea, fatigue, restlessness, and calcification of the soft tissues of the lungs and the kidneys, as well as the bones. There is evidence that the synthetic active forms of vitamin D may be a better treatment in individuals with malabsorption since smaller doses can be used, and so decrease the risk of toxicity. These forms also act much more quickly to reverse deficiency symptoms.

Chapter 8

VITAMIN E

Recent vitamin E studies suggest that this vitamin plays a vital role in the biological functions related to aging. While vitamin E may not necessarily cause anyone to live longer, there are indications that it may slow down the aging process and prevent premature aging by prolonging the useful life of our cells, thus maintaining the function of our organs. For example, studies have shown that red blood cells of normal people who received vitamin E supplements aged far less than the cells of those who received no supplements. Human cells grown in a medium enriched with extra amounts of vitamin E divided and lived much longer than cells grown in ordinary culture mediums. Further studies are needed, but the results of such experiments do indicate exciting possibilities.

What holds true for the cells in these experiments may hold true for other cells of the body, since vitamin E is utilized by practically all of our tissues. The bulk of it is stored in the muscles and fat tissue, but the highest concentrations are in the pituitary gland, adrenal gland, and testes. In animal studies, vitamin E deficiency has been implicated in widely diverse conditions including cataracts, muscular and neuromuscular disease, and in the weakening of the cells of the lungs, liver, heart, and blood. It also causes testicular degeneration and sterility in animals, which has resulted in vitamin E's reputed powers to improve your sex life. Although vitamin E *is* highly concentrated in the testes, its reputation as a "sex vitamin" has never been established in humans.

Much of vitamin E's usefulness seems to stem from its ability as a powerful antioxidant (see Chapter 3) and anticarcinogen. There is a large body of evidence to support this role as well as the synergism of vitamin E with selenium, another antioxidant. Part of vitamin E's benefits may be due to its ability to protect vitamins A and C from oxidation, thus keeping them potent. In addition, vitamin E helps to increase the level of superoxide dismutase, an enzyme produced in our own bodies which is a powerful free radical scavenger. Vitamin E is also able to prevent oxidation of polyunsaturated fats (PUFA) and maintain the strength and healthy functioning of our cells' membranes. Oxidation occurs when carcinogens react with PUFA in our bodies, forming free radicals and peroxides which damage our cells. This ability to protect our cells from the harmful effects of these toxic substances has far-reaching implications in relation to aging and the development of many degenerative diseases such as cancer. However, because these are subtle changes that occur in individual cells, they are difficult to detect until it is too late.

In addition to its antioxidant capabilities, vitamin E protects the body against a variety of carcinogens and toxins—including mercury, lead, carbon tetrachloride, benzene, ozone, and nitrous oxide. It prevents the formation of nitrosamines from nitrites and nitrates found in cured meats, cigarette smoke, and polluted air. Several studies on vitamin E and cancer have shown that lower levels of this vitamin are indeed associated with an increased risk for lung cancer, colorectal cancer, and breast cancer. In animals who were exposed to potent carcinogens, it was found that vitamin E reduced the incidence of cancer of the skin, mouth, colon, and breast. Vitamin E has also enhanced the ability of radiation treatments to shrink implanted cancerous tumors in animals. In addition, there is evidence that vitamin E may protect cancer chemotherapy patients from some of the anticancer drugs' damaging effects on normal cells, but not on cancer cells, thus reducing some of the drugs' side effects without reducing their effectiveness.

The studies that have been done on vitamin E and the circulation have yielded tantalizing results, but remain for the most part inconclusive or conflicting. However, I and other practitioners have found that vitamin E does improve blood flow to the extremities. Some practitioners have reported positive results in treating circulatory problems such as angina, arteriosclerosis, and thrombophlebitis. Others have reported that supplementation improves the symptoms in some people with intermittent claudication (poor blood circulation to the legs), causing attacks of muscle weakness and pain. This condition is often found in the elderly and is usually treated with drugs that thin the blood and widen the blood vessels to encourage the blood to flow more easily. Vitamin E may relieve the condition through the same mechanisms, without the accompanying side effects.

Some data indicate that vitamin E has the ability to increase the level of high-density lipoproteins (HDLs) in men and women with initially low levels of this substance. HDL is a form of cholesterol recently discovered to be very protective against heart disease. Some studies have also shown that vitamin E lowers cholesterol levels in the blood. It may also prevent cholesterol and platelets from clogging the arteries. In several studies it was suggested that vitamin E plays an important role in the metabolism of fats in the arterial wall.

Some studies have shown that vitamin E helps lessen fibrocystic breast disease (benign lumps in the breast). In one study, 85 percent of the supplemented group responded to treatment, with total disappearance of cysts and tenderness in 38 percent of the patients. My patients with fibrocystic disease have responded beautifully when vitamin E supplements were included in their health program.

Vitamin E may play a role in the healing of wounds and in the reduction of scar formation. Although no conclusive studies have been done to date, many practitioners including myself recommend vitamin E to prevent scar formation. Some physicians prescribe vitamin E to lessen the risk of internal scar formation which leads to hardening of the implants used in surgery for breast augmentation. Others recommend puncturing vitamin E capsules and applying the oil topically *after a scab has formed* to promote healing and reduce scarring.

Animal studies have clearly shown that excesses of vitamin E have a beneficial effect on resistance to disease. A small human study of people with an autoimmune disease called discoid lupus erythematosus showed that large doses of vitamin E had a beneficial effect. Patients suffering from rheumatoid arthritis, another autoimmune disease, have also benefited from vitamin E supplementation. In a study of seven patients who were given vitamin E and selenium, along with their usual treatment which had become no longer effective, joint pain either diminished or disappeared completely.

Vitamin E may be important for normal functioning of the nervous system. Certain children with progressive neuromuscular disease were shown to have a vitamin E deficiency. Their symptoms, which included difficulty walking, frequent falling, and abnormal reflexes, improved after vitamin E supplementation.

Vitamin E helps alleviate the symptoms associated with premenstrual syndrome (PMS). Many of my female patients have enjoyed marked improvement in their PMS symptoms in as short a period of time as two months. Studies also indicate that vitamin E supplementation may be useful for treating excess bleeding due to insertion of an intrauterine device, and for lipofusin ("age" or "liver" spots). I have also had excellent results using vitamin E supplementation in menopausal women to reduce "hot flashes." Vitamin E has been shown to reduce the incidence of breast cancers in experimental animals and enhanced the therapeutic effectiveness of radiation on breast cancer.

Classical vitamin E deficiency symptoms include the premature aging and death of red blood cells (leading to anemia), neurological disturbances such as difficulty in walking, and fragile capillaries. These symptoms generally appear only when there is the severe fat malabsorption that occurs in people with disorders of the pancreas, tropical sprue, celiac disease, cystic fibrosis, and in premature infants. Vitamin E–deficient premature infants may also suffer from disorders of the retina, which can lead to blindness. The RDA to prevent these overt deficiencies is approximately 7–13 milligrams (10–20 IU) for men and women.

New data suggest that many other people (that is, without severe fat malabsorption) are at risk for prolonged marginal vitamin E intake which may influence aging, cancer, and heart disease. In recent years, we've all been told to reduce our consumption of saturated fats such as butter and increase our consumption of polyunsaturated fats such as vegetable oil and margarine. This increase in PUFA is supposed to reduce the risk of coronary disease, but it also increases our need for protective vitamin E. Since the vegetable oils that are high in PUFA are also naturally high in protective vitamin E, this would seem to pose no problem. However, *most of the commercial polyunsaturated oils are so highly processed, there is very little vitamin E left.* So while we are increasing our PUFA consumption, we are not correspondingly increasing our vitamin E, a situation that has many implications. For example, some studies have suggested that people who ingest high amounts of processed polyunsaturated vegetable oils with inadequate amounts of vitamin E may have a higher cancer risk, particularly breast cancer.

Food Sources: Vitamin E generally occurs in the fats of vegetable foods. Natural vegetable oils are a particularly rich source of vitamin E, with cottonseed, corn, soybean, safflower, and wheat germ oil having the highest concentrations. Smaller amounts of vitamin E are found in whole grains, dark green leafy vegetables, nuts, and legumes. Animal foods such as meat and dairy products have some vitamin E, but generally are low in this nutrient.

Cooking and processing causes foods to lose their vitamin E since it is destroyed by heat, alkali, light, air, and freezing. The milling of grains, for example, causes them to lose about 80 percent of their vitamin E. As mentioned earlier, commercially processed vegetable oils are low in vitamin E. In fact, the by-products of processed oils have become important sources for the production of vitamin E supplements used by humans and animals! If you depend on vegetable oils for your vitamin E, choose cold-pressed or unrefined oils.

OPTIMUM DAILY ALLOWANCE—ODA

For optimum general health, the basic Optimum Daily Allowance for vitamin E is:

200–800 IU for men and women

In my clinical experience, I have found the following amounts of vitamin E to be valuable for:

Cancer prevention	400–800 IU
Cardiovascular disease prevention	400–800 IU
Poor circulation	600–1200 IU
Wound healing	400–800 IU
Aging	400–800 IU
Fibrocystic breast disease	400–800 IU
Premenstrual syndrome	400–800 IU
Prevention of excessive bleeding with intrauterine devices	100–400 IU
Menopausal "hot flashes"	400–800 IU

Remember: If you have a medical condition, please consult your physician before taking supplements.

Warning: If you have high blood pressure, you should not take large amounts of vitamin E unless you are being monitored by a professional. At the onset of vitamin therapy, the blood pressure may actually rise temporarily. In addition, you should start with a low dose of 100 IU and increase it gradually. If you are on anticoagulants, do not take large amounts of vitamin E (over 400 IU daily) without professional supervision.

SUPPLEMENTS

Vitamin E actually consists of four substances: alpha, beta, delta, and gamma tocopherol. There are natural and synthetic forms of all the tocopherols. The naturally occurring form of vitamin E is the "D" form, as in D-alpha tocopherol. The synthetic form is the "DL" form, as in DL-alpha tocopherol. The natural form appears to be the most absorbable; however, it is also the most expensive. For my budget-conscious patients, I recommend a supplement that contains a combination of D and DL as a good compromise.

Vitamin E supplements often contain alpha alone, because that has been shown to be the most active form. However, I recommend that you buy your tocopherols "mixed" since that is how they exist in food.

Vitamin E succinate is a synthetic vitamin and comes in a dry, oil-free powder. Since it is the least absorbable form of vitamin E in normal individuals, I recommend it only if you have a problem with fat malabsorption.

TOXICITY AND ADVERSE EFFECTS

There is no well-documented toxicity of vitamin E in doses of up to 800–1200 IU per day. However, with very high doses (over 1200 IU per day), some adverse effects such as nausea, flatulence, diarrhea, headache, heart palpitations, and fainting have been reported. These are completely reversible upon reduction of the dosage. You should begin with a lower dose of vitamin E and increase the dosage gradually to minimize the possibility of adverse effects.

Chapter 9

VITAMIN K

Vitamin K is found in food, but is also created by the bacteria in our intestines, and so is not strictly a vitamin.

Vitamin K's most important function is the role it plays in the production of coagulation (blood clotting) factors in the body. It interacts with a substance called prothrombin, which is then converted to thrombin. This in turn converts fibrinogen to fibrin, which is what creates the blood clot. (By the way, many rodent poisons work because they are actually counteract vitamin K, which causes rodents to bleed to death.)

Recent studies have revealed other possible roles for vitamin K. For example, low levels of vitamin K may be related to the development of osteoporosis, and may also affect behavior.

Food Sources: Vitamin K is distributed fairly widely in food, with the following containing the highest amounts: spinach, green cabbage, tomatoes, liver, and lean meat. There are also appreciable amounts in egg yolk, whole wheat, and strawberries.

OPTIMUM DAILY ALLOWANCE—ODA

There is no Recommended Daily Allowance (RDA) or Optimum Daily Allowance (ODA) of vitamin K. Since it is so easily available from the diet and synthesized in the body, deficiencies in vitamin K are rare, and usually only occur when there is malabsorption due to bowel obstruction, sprue, bowel shunts, regional ileitis and ulcerative colitis, or chronic liver disease. Vitamin K is given prophylactically to infants at birth to prevent hemorrhage, and presurgically to those people who have bleeding and clotting disorders.

Remember: If you have a medical condition, please consult with your physician before taking supplements, especially if you are on anticoagulant therapy.

SUPPLEMENTS

Vitamin K is a general term used to describe a group of similar compounds including K-1 (from plants), K-2 (made by our intestinal bacteria), and K-3 (synthetic). Since vitamin K is widely available in foods and made in our bodies, supplements are necessary only with malabsorption or medical disorders. Please consult with your physician before taking vitamin K supplements, especially if you are on anticoagulant therapy.

TOXICITY AND ADVERSE EFFECTS

The major symptom of too much vitamin K is hemolytic anemia, where the red blood cells die more quickly than usual and the body is unable to replace them.

WATER-SOLUBLE VITAMINS

Chapter 10

VITAMIN B COMPLEX

The vitamins that belong in this group are B-1 (thiamin), B-2 (riboflavin), B-3 (niacin and niacinamide), B-6 (pyridoxine), B-12 (cobalamin), folic acid, pantothenic acid, biotin, choline, inositol, and PABA.

The term "B complex" is somewhat of a misnomer in that each B vitamin has its own unique biological role to play and its own individual properties. However, as a group they do have so much in common that they are often thought of as a single entity. In addition, the B vitamins work together in the body and many of them are found in the same foods.

This chapter will give you an overview of the group of vitamins known as B complex. It will provide you with a general understanding of their uses, sources, RDAs and ODAs. The following chapters will then deal with each B vitamin individually.

The B vitamins are utilized as coenzymes in almost all parts of the body. They are essential for maintaining healthy nerves, skin, hair, eyes, liver, and mouth, and good muscle tone in the gastrointestinal tract. The B vitamins give us energy, being necessary for the metabolism of carbohydrates, fats, and proteins. The traditional RDAs for the B vitamins vary (see following chapters), but in general are quite low—around 2 milligrams each, or less.

Deficiency in a single B vitamin is rare; rather, people tend to have multiple deficiencies, making subtle deficiency symptoms more difficult to diagnose, yet more likely to be present. Researchers have found that activity originally attributed to individual B vitamins actually seems to depend on several acting in concert.

In addition to the well-recognized severe deficiency diseases of the individual B vitamins such as beriberi (thiamin) and pellagra (niacin), new research is turning up other possible clinical deficiencies and uses. For example, the B complex's well-documented involvement with the nervous system has led many practitioners to use high doses of the B vitamins to alleviate psychiatric symptoms such as mild depression, anxiety, nervousness, and poor memory. Vitamin B deficiencies have also been discovered in psychiatric disorders such as schizophrenia, depression, delirium, and anxiety. Some of these patients have responded to B-vitamin supplementation: When it was used to correct a deficiency, these symptoms disappeared. In patients not necessarily deficient in B vitamins, supplementation remains a controversial issue.

Although the B vitamins are not antiaging vitamins per se, they are involved in preventing reactions related to the gradual wear and tear associated with the aging process. B vitamins have also been linked with stress of many kinds. When you are under emotional stress, or undergo surgery, or are sick, pregnant, or breastfeeding, your requirements for the B vitamins automatically go up. And yet it is far from common practice to give hospital patients even low supplemental doses of the B vitamins (or any vitamins).

The B vitamins may play a role in supporting your immune system. According to animal studies, all the B vitamins enhance the immune system in some way if given in excess of the RDA. This is not because B vitamins make white blood cells or antibodies themselves, but because they are involved with the enzymes that make these constituents of our defense system.

Food Sources: Generally, the B vitamins are most plentiful in whole, unrefined grains such as wheat, rice, oats, and rye, and in liver. They are also found in green leafy vegetables, meats, poultry, fish, eggs, nuts, and beans. Most of the B vitamins (and many other nutrients) are removed when grains are highly refined. Although such products may have gone through the so-called "enrichment" process, this replaces only a few nutrients, leaving what was a nicely balanced source of B complex sadly lacking.

TOXICITY AND ADVERSE EFFECTS

In general, there are no known toxicities to the B vitamins.

OPTIMUM DAILY ALLOWANCE—ODA

As you will see from the following chapters on the individual B vitamins, the approximate basic Optimum Daily Allowance for B complex is:

50–300 mg in men and women (and 25–300 mcg for B-12, folic acid, and biotin)

The entire B complex is generally available in B complex supplements and multivitamin formulas. If you buy a "B complex 50" for example, it usually contains 50 milligrams of all the B vitamins measured in milligrams (B-1, B-2, B-3, B-6, choline, inositol, and PABA) and 50 micrograms of all those measured in micrograms (B-12, folic acid, and biotin).

There are many physicians and other practitioners who may give as much as 2000 milligrams (or micrograms) of a B vitamin. However, it is not recommended that you take this amount without professional supervision. If you have a medical condition, do not take any amount without consulting your physician.

The ratio of one B vitamin to another in supplements is generally 1:1. *Never take high doses of a single B vitamin without increasing the amount you take of all the others.* This is not only because the B vitamins tend to work together. It is also because B vitamins compete in the intestines for absorption by the body; if you take in an enormous amount of B-1, for instance, you might decrease the amount of B-3 absorbed and ironically wind up with a B vitamin imbalance. Many well-meaning but insufficiently educated professionals mistakenly prescribe supplements of a single member of the B vitamin complex to their patients. For example, professionals have often prescribed B-6 to their patients for carpal tunnel syndrome. Some of the side effects ascribed to B-6 supplementation (see Chapter 14) may be due to the fact that other B vitamins were not given along with the B-6. In my opinion, a severe imbalance of the other B vitamins may have been the actual cause of the observed side effects of massive doses (2000 milligrams) of B-6.

To simplify matters, many people buy a B-complex or multivitamin supplement that contains all the B vitamins. Once you have established your basic ODA of the B vitamins, you can then add additional amounts of one or two individual B vitamins to suit your particular needs. In general, it is safe to take up to about two to three times the amount of the other B's you are taking. For instance, if you take 100 milligrams of the entire B complex, you can then safely take a total of up to 200–300 milligrams of vitamin B-6.

SUPPLEMENTS

B-complex is widely available as a supplement. Individual supplements of each B vitamin are also available. Brewer's yeast is a low-potency food supplement for a variety of B vitamins.

Chapter 11

VITAMIN B-1 (THIAMIN)

Vitamin B-1, also known as thiamin, plays an essential role in the metabolism of carbohydrates in the body. Since the cells of the nervous system are extremely sensitive to carbohydrate metabolism, this may be why the brain and the nerves are the first to show signs of thiamin deficiency. Thiamin is also involved in converting fatty acids into steroids in the body. It is necessary for proper growth and for the maintenance of healthy skin. There is some indication that thiamin, like all the B vitamins, plays a role in our resistance to disease. Vitamin B-1 is also looked upon as an antioxidant and may decrease oxidation of lipids (fats) in the body.

Since thiamin is needed as a catalyst in burning carbohydrates in the body, it should come as no surprise that if you increase your daily intake of either complex or simple carbohydrate calories, your need for thiamin increases because the extra carbohydrates utilize more vitamin B-1. This affects both junk-food junkies and health-conscious people who have switched to high complex-carbohydrate diets.

Thiamin requirements also go up during periods of increased metabolism. These include fever, muscular activity, an overactive thyroid, pregnancy, lactation, and perhaps during all forms of physical and emotional stress. In one study, patients undergoing surgery showed a significant fall in their thiamin levels forty-eight hours after the surgery, indicating a higher rate of use. Oral contraceptives have been found to lower body levels of thiamin. Kidney patients undergoing long-term dialysis and patients being fed intravenously are at risk of becoming thiamin deficient. Drinking large amounts of tea and coffee (whether decaffeinated or not) hinders thiamin absorption and therefore also increases the risk of deficiency. In fact, it is possible for heavy tea or coffee drinkers to have nervous symptoms associated with thiamin deficiency and be misdiagnosed or not seek medical help. Other foods with antithiamin activity are blueberries, red chicory, black currants, brussels sprouts, and red cabbage.

(Ascorbic acid, however, has been shown to protect against thiamin destruction in some of these foods.)

The classical deficiency disease for B-1 is beriberi, a disease which affects the gastrointestinal, cardiovascular, and peripheral nervous system. Advanced symptoms are indigestion, constipation, headaches, insomnia, a heaviness and weakness in the legs often followed by cramping of leg muscles, burning and numbness of feet; in addition, the heart may become damaged or enlarged, or beat rapidly and irregularly. Severe vitamin B-1 deficiency also causes Korsakoff's syndrome (confusion, loss of memory, delusions, amnesia), and Wernickes disease (apathy, confusion, delirium). To prevent these symptoms of severe thiamin deficiency, the RDA for vitamin B-1 is 1.4 milligrams for males, and 1.1 milligrams for females (slightly higher if pregnant or lactating).

In this country, beriberi is usually confined to alcoholics. However, as we have seen, there are many other groups of people who are at risk of being deficient in this nutrient to a lesser extent and so suffer more subtle effects on the nervous system, digestive system, and heart. As a result, many people may in fact be experiencing early, subclinical symptoms of beriberi including fatigue, apathy, mental confusion, inability to concentrate, poor memory, insomnia, anorexia (loss of appetite), loss of weight and strength, emotional instability, irritability, depression, irrational anger and fear.

In addition, it has been discovered that schizophrenics tend to be particularly low in thiamin. A recent survey of psychiatric patients showed 47 percent to be deficient in at least one of three vitamins assessed. Thiamin deficiency was detected in 30 percent of the patients; however, only *one* patient showed clinical symptoms of deficiency. In the mentally ill, the elderly, and people with poor diets, subclinical thiamin deficiency is common. Conversely, inadequate intake of vitamins, particularly of B-1, may result in mental illness. Some psychiatrists use B-1 in combination with other B vitamins for various emotional and psychiatric illnesses, oftentimes with medication. There is some evidence that B-1 is of value to cancer patients to prevent the cell damage associated with the disease.

Food Sources: The richest sources for thiamin are organ meats (especially liver), pork, dried beans, peas, soybeans, peanuts, whole grains such as whole wheat bread, brown rice, wheat germ, rice bran, egg yolks, poultry, and fish. Medium sources include plums, dried prunes, raisins, asparagus, beans, broccoli, oatmeal, brussels sprouts, and a wide variety of nuts. In addition, many foods are fortified with this vitamin to prevent overt deficiency symptoms. Foods lose their thiamin content if exposed to ultraviolet light, sulfites, nitrites, and live yeast. When bread is baked, the flour's thiamin content is reduced by 15–20 percent; broiling and roasting meat reduces thiamin by 25 percent; and boiling meat by 50 percent. Vitamin B-1 is also destroyed by thiaminase, which is contained in raw fish.

OPTIMUM DAILY ALLOWANCE—ODA

For optimum general health, the basic Optimum Daily Allowance for thiamin is:

25–300 mg for men and women

In my clinical experience, I have found the following amounts of thiamin to be valuable for:

Anxiety, depression . . . . 100–500 mg
High complex carbohydrate diet . . . . 50–100 mg
Emotional or physical stress . . . . 100–500 mg

Remember: If you have a medical condition or psychiatric disorder, please consult with your physician before taking supplements.

SUPPLEMENTS

B-1 (as thiamin hydrochloride and thiamin mononitrate) is available in individual supplements and in B complex supplements in a wide range of potencies.

TOXICITY AND ADVERSE EFFECTS

Riboflavin has no known toxicity.

Chapter 12

VITAMIN B-2
(RIBOFLAVIN)

Vitamin B-2 is also known as riboflavin. It is involved in two types of energy metabolism: in protein metabolism to form enzymes necessary to transport oxygen to the cells; and in metabolism of lipids such as fatty acids. This may explain why riboflavin-deficient people tend to tire easily and have a poor appetite, perhaps with some digestive disturbances.

Riboflavin is needed for tissue repair and many types of physical stress have been associated with an increased need for this vitamin. These include burns, injuries, surgery, tuberculosis, fever, congestive heart failure, malignancies, hypothyroidism, acute diabetes, and alcoholism.

The blood requires riboflavin: There is a vitamin B-2 anemia, perhaps because a deficiency inhibits red blood cell production, or because it causes them to die too early. There is evidence that riboflavin may work in conjunction with iron to correct iron-deficiency anemia. Researchers have discovered that some sickle-cell anemia patients were deficient in B-2 and may have an increased need of this vitamin. Riboflavin may play a role in our defense system, since animal studies have indicated that riboflavin deficiency reduces their ability to produce antibodies. Animal experimentation also suggests that riboflavin deficiency may increase the susceptibility of the tissue of the esophagus to cancer.

Riboflavin is essential for healthy eyes. Since it is found in the pigment of the retina, this vitamin is needed for the eyes to adapt to light. B-2 deficiencies can show up as photophobia (excessive sensitivity to light); the eyes may water and become inflamed and bloodshot. Vision may become blurred and the eyes easily tired. Animal studies have shown that there is a correlation between cataracts and a lack of B-2. Many practitioners are beginning to treat the early stages of cataracts in humans with vitamin B-2; their encouraging results may indicate that this vitamin may either prevent cataracts or delay their progress.

As with B-1 and the other B vitamins, B-2 is sometimes given (often-times along with medication) to patients with psychiatric disorders, since its deficiency has been discovered in this population. Another indication that B-2 is useful for neurological problems is its beneficial effect on carpal tunnel syndrome. I and other practitioners have had marvelous results when we give B-2, along with B-6, to patients with this painful neurological disease affecting the hands.

The classical deficiency symptoms of vitamin B-2 involve the lips, tongue, eyes, skin, and nervous system. Early signs of deficiency include changes in the eyes such as increased light sensitivity, tearing, burning and itching, eye fatigue, and decrease in the sharpness of vision. Cheilosis (tiny lesions in the mouth or cracks in the corners of the mouth) is another early warning sign, as are sore or burning lips, inflammation of the tongue, enlarged or purple tongue, and discomfort in eating and swallowing. There may be flaking of the skin around the nose, eyebrows, chin, cheeks, earlobes, or hairline. Dermatitis and sores may also occur on the vulva and scrotum. Behavioral changes are common in B-2 deficiencies, and include depression, moodiness, nervousness, and irritability.

To prevent these overt deficiencies, these are the RDAs for vitamin B-2: 1.4 milligrams in men and 1.1 milligrams in women (slightly higher if pregnant or lactating). Many people may be marginally deficient in B-2 because antibiotics, alcohol, and oral contraceptives may deplete or inter-fere with the absorption or utilization of riboflavin. In addition, exercise may increase the need for B-2, as can being on a weight-loss diet. As we have learned, requirements also go up during any kind of stress, and this includes pregnancy and lactation.

Food Sources: Foods naturally high in B-2 are milk, cheese, yogurt, and eggs; meat, poultry and fish, especially kidney and liver; beans, and spin-ach. Other good sources are avocados, currants, asparagus, broccoli, brus-sels sprouts, and nuts. Unless they are whole-grain, cereals and grains are ordinarily low in riboflavin; however, they are often enriched with B-2. Milk, which is originally a good source of B-2, loses 10 to 12 percent of this nutrient after it has been pasteurized, irradiated for vitamin D, evapo-rated, or dried. Storing it in clear glass bottles leads to losses of up to 75 percent in 3 1/2 hours. Cooking meat causes it to lose about 25 percent of its B-2. Adding sodium bicarbonate to vegetables during cooking (to pre-serve their green color) destroys riboflavin.

OPTIMUM DAILY ALLOWANCE–ODA

To maintain and achieve optimum general health, the basic Optimum Daily Allowance for B-2 is:

50–300 mg for men and women

In my clinical experience, I have found the following amounts of riboflavin to be valuable for:

Stress	50–200 mg
Cataract prevention	100–500 mg
Oral contraceptive use	100–300 mg
Strenuous exercise	50–100 mg
Depression, anxiety	100–500 mg
Carpal tunnel syndrome	100–500 mg (with B-6)

Remember: If you have a medical condition or psychiatric disorder, please consult with your physician before taking supplements.

SUPPLEMENTS

Riboflavin is available in many potencies, both individually and in B-complex supplements.

TOXICITY AND ADVERSE EFFECTS

Riboflavin has no known toxicity.

Chapter 13

VITAMIN B-3
(NIACIN AND NIACINAMIDE)

Vitamin B-3 comes in two forms: niacin (or nicotinic acid) and niacinamide. Our bodies can make niacinamide from tryptophan, an amino acid found in animal foods, but this accounts for only a small fraction of our needs. We also convert niacin into niacinamide. Vitamin B-3 is a coenzyme in several important biochemical functions, particularly those needed to maintain a healthy skin, gastrointestinal tract, and nervous system.

Vitamin B-3 is also used by the body in the metabolism of lipids. Much of the current excitement about B-3 surrounds the use of niacin (not niacinamide) in treating high levels of cholesterol. An overwhelming number of studies have shown that niacin is effective in reducing both cholesterol and triglyceride levels in the blood. For example, one study compared the efficacy of niacin with that of clofibrate, a widely prescribed drug that lowers cholesterol. Niacin was much more effective than the drug in lowering serum cholesterol, VLDL, and triglycerides. It also significantly increased HDL cholesterol. In this and other studies, the authors conclude that because of these effects, especially when combined with niacin's low cost and low toxicity, niacin should be considered the treatment of choice in many patients with elevated cholesterol levels. Other agents used to treat this condition have some serious side effects, such as higher incidence of gastrointestinal cancer and increased risk of gallbladder disease. In my clinical practice I have found niacin to be extremely effective in lowering cholesterol and triglycerides. When these patients returned to their physicians for follow-up exams, they were delighted with the results. When I gave one particular patient niacin supplements as part of his overall health program, he was able to reduce his cholesterol from 350 to 225 and his triglycerides from 225 to 90.

Early symptoms of niacin deficiency that appear in the nervous system are apprehension, irritability, depression, weakness, and loss of memory. These may be followed by disorientation, confusion, and hysteria. Therefore many practitioners use niacin and/or niacinamide alone or in conjunction with other medications in the treatment of mental disorders such as anxiety, nervousness, depression, and even schizophrenia; this use, however, is still controversial. Studies have suggested that niacinamide (as well as vitamins E, B-6, and calcium pantothenate) may be useful in the treatment of epilepsy together with anticonvulsants.

B-3, in the form of niacin, is a vasodilator. Since vasodilators widen the blood vessels and increase the blood flow to the extremities, niacin is used for various circulatory problems.

In addition, it appears from several studies that niacinamide is effective against more than one type of carcinogen and so may be useful in preventing several types of cancer.

Severe niacin deficiency is a major factor in the development of the disease of pellagra, which is characterized by "the three D's": dermatitis, diarrhea, and dementia. In order to prevent these deficiency symptoms, the Recommended Daily Allowance for vitamin B-3 is 18–19 milligrams for men, and 14–15 milligrams for women (an additional 2 milligrams is recommended for pregnant women; an additional 5 milligrams for lactating women). Easily observable deficiencies of this vitamin generally occur only in alcoholics and other severely malnourished people. Niacin deficiency is also quite common in people who eat corn-based diets because the niacin contained in the corn is unabsorbable. (The exception is in Mexico, where they soak corn in lime water, which releases the niacin.) B-3 requirements may be higher in people who have cancer, people who are being treated with the drug isoniazid (for tuberculosis), women who take oral contraceptives, and people who have protein deficiencies.

Food Sources: Vitamin B-3 is found in meat (beef, pork), fish, milk and cheese, whole wheat, potatoes, corn flour, eggs, broccoli, tomatoes, and carrots. However, it is often present in the food in a form which is not absorbable. Since B-3 may be lost in the cooking water, it is advisable to steam, bake, or stir-fry vegetables to spare as much of this vitamin as possible.

OPTIMUM DAILY ALLOWANCE—ODA

For optimum general health, the basic Optimum Daily Allowance for niacin, niacinamide, or a combination of both is:

25–300 mg for men and women

(You may wish to take 10–25 percent of your total B-3 intake as niacin.)

In my clinical experience, I have found the following amounts of B-3 to be valuable for:

Anxiety or depression	100–500 mg niacin or niacinamide (under professional advice)
Circulatory problems	50–500 mg niacin
High triglycerides and/or cholesterol	50–500 mg niacin (up to 2000 mg under professional advice)

Remember: If you have a medical condition or psychiatric symptoms, please consult with your physician before taking supplements.

SUPPLEMENTS

Both niacin and niacinamide are widely available as supplements. I recommend niacin rather than niacinamide for circulatory problems and for lowering cholesterol and triglycerides.

TOXICITY AND ADVERSE EFFECTS

The only adverse effect of niacin supplementation is a flush, which makes you turn red and perhaps slightly itchy. High doses of niacin may exacerbate a pre-existing gastric or duodenal ulcer. If you have a history of an ulcer, please consult with a professional before taking large doses.

Taking niacin after a meal or taking an aspirin an hour before you take the niacin will lessen or prevent the flush without losing the beneficial effect.

There is no known toxicity to this vitamin, except with very high doses. Very high doses of niacin (2000 milligrams per day or more) have been shown to have adverse effects on the liver; these effects are reversible when the supplementation is stopped. In addition, oftentimes the body adjusts to the high dosage of niacin and the liver no longer shows signs of toxicity. This high intake should be monitored by a trained professional.

Chapter 14

VITAMIN B-6 (PYRIDOXINE)

Vitamin B-6, also known as pyridoxine, is one of the most essential, widely utilized vitamins in the body. It is a coenzyme which participates in over sixty enzymatic reactions involved in the metabolism of amino acids (the building blocks of protein) and of essential fatty acids. It is therefore needed for the proper growth and maintenance of almost all our body functions. Its deficiency has been found to bring about an astonishing variety of symptoms.

The most frequently diagnosed and well-recognized deficiency symptoms of vitamin B-6 occur in the skin and nervous system. The changes in the skin and mucous membranes are similar to those caused by other members of the B-complex group. These include seborrheic dermatitis (particularly around the nose, eyes, eyebrows, the skin behind the ears, and the mouth), acne, cheilosis and stomatitis (tiny sores and cracks in and around the mouth), and glossitis (inflamed tongue).

The nervous system is dependent on B-6 in a variety of ways. Too little of this vitamin is associated with problems such as depression, confusion, dizziness, insomnia, irritability, nervousness, a pins and needles feeling in the hands and feet, even brain wave abnormalities and convulsions. Vitamin B-6 is necessary for the production of serotonin and other neurotransmitters in the brain, and there is evidence that depressed patients have disorders in the production of serotonin. Although "megavitamin" therapy for psychiatric symptoms is controversial, the results of many studies indicate an association between B-6 deficiency and emotional illness including depression and schizophrenia. I and many other practitioners feel that there is enough evidence to warrant its use as an alternative treatment when psychotropic drugs fail or result in toxicity. Others suggest it be used along with psychotropic drugs.

Recent research shows that B-6 may have a much greater effect on the nervous system than previously thought. For example, a number of recent studies report that patients with carpal tunnel syndrome (a neurological condition that causes swelling and nerve compression in the wrist, leading to weakness, pain, burning, numbness or tingling in the hand) respond to B-6 supplementation, especially when combined with B-2. In addition, infants fed formulas low in vitamin B-6 have suffered epileptic-like convulsions, weight loss, nervous irritability, and stomach problems. These problems and other forms of childhood epilepsy respond to B-6 supplements. Autistic children also have been shown to improve when given B-6 along with magnesium.

B-6 is important for women who suffer from PMS (premenstrual syndrome), which may include some or all of the following symptoms: depression, irritability, tiredness, painful and swollen breasts, bloated abdomen, swollen fingers and ankles, headache, stomachache, and backache. Many studies have shown that B-6 reduces or eliminates these symptoms for most women. We don't know why, but it may be because high estrogen levels after ovulation result in an increased need for B-6 or a decreased ability to absorb it. In addition, B-6 tends to act as a natural diuretic and this would also help reduce PMS symptoms. At any rate, I have seen remarkable results in my own patients and many researchers suggest B-6 as the first line of treatment for this syndrome, before progesterone is considered.

A number of studies have shown that women who take oral contraceptives tend to have lower blood levels of this vitamin. This may be responsible for the lethargy, fatigue, and mental depression experienced by some women on oral contraceptives, since B-6 supplementation improves these symptoms.

B-6 is of special concern for both pregnant and lactating women, as studies have shown the requirement goes up at these times. However, these women may not be getting enough: One study found that women consumed only 50 percent of the RDA during the last month of pregnancy, and breastfeeding women consumed only 60 percent of the RDA after delivery. These figures are of special concern not only for the mother, but for her infant too. It has been found, for instance, that B-6 supplementation can reduce or cure the nausea and vomiting of pregnancy. Another study found that Apgar scores were significantly better for infants of mothers who took several times the RDA of B-6 than those who took close to the RDA. (Apgar scores are taken soon after birth and are a predictor of general health and well-being.) Adequate levels of B-6 are also of importance in lactating women because of the previously mentioned association of B-6 deficiency with convulsions and irritability in some infants.

Vitamin B-6 is needed for healthy blood and blood vessels. It is required by the body to turn iron into hemoglobin, and to produce red blood cells and antibodies. A deficiency can therefore cause anemia and a depression in the immune responses of the body. Studies also indicate that vitamin B-6 may help prevent arteriosclerosis.

Asthmatics may benefit from B-6 supplementation, as may those with sickle-cell anemia, diabetes, and "Chinese Restaurant Syndrome" (an adverse reaction to MSG, the symptoms of which include a burning sensation and pressure of the face, chest pain, headache, lightheadedness, and heartburn). Pyridoxine has been shown to be of use in the treatment of recurring oxalate kidney stones in adults, and in kidney failure in some infants. Experiments with animals suggest a diet deficient in B-6 may be involved in premature aging. Another experiment suggests that B-6 holds promise as a treatment for melanoma, a deadly form of cancer.

The list of benefits and uses of B-6 is a long one, but it is difficult for men and women to obtain even their respective RDAs of 2.2 milligrams and 2 milligrams from food. Certain groups in the population such as women, dieters, adolescent girls, alcoholics, and the elderly have consistently been found to take in less than the RDA. For example, one study of seventy-four female college students (excluding those taking oral contraceptives) found that only one of them was getting the full RDA of B-6. In addition, many people may require more than the RDA. Among the situations that raise the B-6 requirement are: exposure to radiation; certain drugs including oral contraceptives, isoniazid, penicillamine, semicarbazide, and cycloserine; tobacco and air pollutants; cardiac failure; and of course stress.

Food Sources: All foods contain small amounts of B-6. The following foods are thought to be the highest: eggs, fish, spinach, carrots, peas, meat, chicken, fish (especially herring and salmon), brewer's yeast, walnuts, sunflower seeds, and wheat germ. Medium sources include brown rice and other whole grains, blackstrap molasses, avocado, cantaloupe, bananas, cabbage, and beans.

However, it has recently been discovered that data on the vitamin B-6 content of foods is unreliable, since the amount of B-6 in foods does not necessarily represent the amount of the vitamin that is actually available to humans. This is true to some degree of all nutrients, but studies have shown that the bioavailability of the B-6 content of foods may in fact be quite limited. In addition, the content of B-6 in foods is affected by heat, oxygen and light. Up to 70 percent of the B-6 in foods may be lost during cooking, processing, and refining.

OPTIMUM DAILY ALLOWANCE—ODA

For optimum general health, the basic Optimum Daily Allowance for vitamin B-6 is:

25–300 mg for men and women

In my clinical experience, I have found the following amounts of B-6 to be valuable for:

Kidney stones (oxalate)	100–300 mg
As a diuretic	100–300 mg
Premenstrual syndrome	50–300 mg
Depression and anxiety	100–500 mg
Oral contraceptive use	50–300 mg
Carpal tunnel syndrome	50–500 mg
Asthma	50–300 mg

Remember: If you have a medical condition or psychiatric symptoms, please consult with your physician before taking supplements. High doses of B-6 should not be used in people who are being treated with Levodopa for Parkinson's Disease.

SUPPLEMENTS

Vitamin B-6 is available as pyridoxine hydrochloride (the most commonly available) and pyridoxine 5 phosphate (which may possibly be better absorbed). Both forms have been shown to be equally active in experimental animals, which leads us to believe that they act similarly in humans also.

TOXICITY AND ADVERSE EFFECTS

B-6 is relatively nontoxic, but some problems with the nervous system have been reported. This only occurs with huge doses of 2000–6000 milligrams of B-6 daily, although there are isolated cases of toxicity with smaller doses. These side effects appear to be reversible when the dosage is discontinued. In addition, dependency has been induced in normal adults who were given 200 milligrams daily for thirty-three days; this results in a deficiency when supplementation is stopped abruptly.

Chapter 15

VITAMIN B-12
(COBALAMIN)

Vitamin B-12, also known as cobalamin, is a coenzyme needed for fat and carbohydrate metabolism. The classic deficiency disease of B-12 is pernicious anemia, with symptoms of pallor and fatigue. This type of anemia is rather common and appears most frequently in alcoholics, the elderly, and in strict vegetarians (non–lacto-ovo). It is imperative to use diagnostic tests to distinguish B-12 anemia from folic acid anemia. If folic acid is given someone already deficient in B-12, severe B-12 deficiency will develop.

Vitamin B-12 deficiencies have been diagnosed in people with any one of a wide variety of gastrointestinal problems. For example, there may be a deficiency of "intrinsic factor"—a constituent of gastric juice required for the absorption of this vitamin, or a bacterial or parasitic infection, or sprue (the inability to digest the gluten present in grains such as wheat and rye).

Vitamin B-12 is involved in the production of myelin, which is the sheath that covers our nerves. Therefore the association between B-12 deficiency and an impaired nervous system function is well established. B-12 deficiency may play a part in many mild to severe physical and emotional symptoms such as confusion, moodiness, memory loss, peripheral neuritis, leg and finger incoordination, depression, and psychosis. These can occur even when there are no signs of changes in the blood to indicate either low levels of B-12 or anemia.

Recent studies have uncovered a possible link between Alzheimer-type dementia and low vitamin B-12 levels in the blood. Although it is not known whether there is a direct causal relationship, it may be that prolonged low blood levels of B-12 produce the irreversible neurological changes seen in this disease.

In addition, vitamin B-12, when combined with ascorbic acid, has been shown to inhibit the formation of cancer in laboratory mice. Prolonged excess exposure to nitrous oxide ("laughing gas") may result in lowered blood levels of this vitamin. Early studies suggested that vitamin C supplementation may destroy B-12 in the body. Subsequent studies using improved technology have shown that large doses of vitamin C do not have this effect. On the contrary, the absorption of the cyanocobalamin form of B-12 is slightly increased in the presence of vitamin C.

The RDA for vitamin B-12 is 3 micrograms for men and women. Although we have the ability to produce B-12 in the intestines, we are not sure how much of this can be absorbed by the body.

Food Sources: Generally, the amount of B-12 in foods is small. Most sources are animal in origin: lamb and beef kidneys, lamb, beef, calf, and pork livers are the highest in B-12. Good sources are beef, herring, and mackerel. Egg yolk, milk, cheese, clams, sardines, salmon, crab, and oysters also have reasonable amounts. It was recently discovered that some fermented foods, such as tofu, contain appreciable amounts of B-12.

Vitamin B-12 is not stable in the presence of heat, acid, or light, and is susceptible to oxidation, so care is required during the storage and cooking of foods.

OPTIMUM DAILY ALLOWANCE—ODA

For optimum general health, the basic Optimum Daily Allowance for vitamin B-12 is:

25–300 mcg for men and women

In my clinical experience, I have found the following amounts of B-12 to be valuable for:

Anxiety or depression . . . . . . 100–500 mcg

B-12 anemia . . . . 250–500 mcg (injections by
your physician may be necessary
if you have malabsorption)

Remember: If you have a medical condition or psychiatric symptoms, please consult with your physician before taking supplements.

SUPPLEMENTS

Cyanocobalamin is the form of B-12 that is most widely used in oral supplements. Hydroxycobalamin is the form of B-12 used in injections; these are recommended if the patient is suffering from B-12 malabsorption.

TOXICITY AND ADVERSE EFFECTS

Vitamin B-12 has no known toxicity.

Chapter 16

FOLIC ACID

Folic acid (also known as folate or folacin) works closely with vitamin B-12 in the body, where it is involved with the metabolism of amino acids and the synthesis of proteins. Since it is needed for the production of RNA and DNA, folate is vital to healthy cell division and replication. Folic acid deficiency affects the tissues that grow or regenerate rapidly, such as the lining of the gastrointestinal tract, the skin, and the bone marrow where blood cells are formed.

Because of the role that folic acid plays in tissue regeneration, there may be an increased need for this nutrient during illness, injury, and surgery, during which time the body repairs itself. It logically follows that folic acid requirements go up during any time of stress.

Studies in humans and in animals have indicated that many aspects of the immune system are affected by a deficiency in folic acid, including the ability to recognize invading microbes and the number and strength of our white blood cells. As a result, inadequate folic acid may render us less resistant to disease.

Folic acid derivatives are coenzymes for neurotransmitters. Recently, some studies have suggested that a folic acid deficiency can produce minor and major mental problems and mood changes including depression, schizophrenia, and dementia. Since large doses of this vitamin have been reported to improve the condition of a certain congenital form of mental retardation, folate may also be connected with other forms of mental retardation or low IQ.

Folate has helped stop or reverse cervical dysplasia in women taking oral contraceptives. Dysplasia is a condition characterized by changes in the structure of the cells. The dysplasia is often suspect as a precancerous condition. If it is severe, surgical removal of the suspicious cells is generally recommended. Evidence suggests that in some women oral contraceptives cause a localized folate deficiency in these cells, somehow making them more susceptible to cancer-causing viruses or chemicals. I have treated many patients whom physicians have referred to my office for this problem. When their physicians gave them follow-up exams, they were delighted to find a reversal of the dysplasia.

Pregnancy may deplete the mother's supply of folic acid because the rapidly growing fetus makes increased demands on her body's stores of this nutrient. This may cause anemia in the mother and birth defects in the child. In one study, mothers of children who were born with harelip were given folic acid prior to and during the first trimester of their next pregnancy. Only one of the supplemented mothers gave birth to another child with harelip; in the unsupplemented group, there were fifteen recurrences. Since oral contraceptives may also affect the level of folate in the blood throughout the body, any woman who goes off the Pill in order to become pregnant should make sure she has adequate folate stored in her body before she conceives.

The need for folic acid is also greater in people who take other kinds of drugs. Studies have shown that aspirin, nitrous oxide as an anesthetic gas, anticonvulsants, sulfasalazine (used for inflammatory bowel disease), trimethropin (used in a diuretic), and methotrexate (an anticancer drug) may interfere with folate absorption or utilization. Therefore, supplementation may be advised while taking these drugs.

The classic deficiency disease of folic acid deficiency is a type of anemia in which the red blood cells are improperly formed; the symptoms include irritability, weakness, sleeping difficulties, and pallor. Diagnostic tests *must* be used to distinguish folic acid anemia from B-12 anemia because giving B-12 to a person already deficient in folic acid will cause severe folic acid deficiency to develop. Classic folic acid deficiency symptoms most often occur in alcoholics and people with intestinal malabsorption usually due to the aging process, gastrointestinal surgery, or some other disease or condition of the digestive system. To prevent overt deficiencies, the RDA of folic acid for men and women is 400 micrograms; 800 micrograms for pregnant women, and 500 micrograms for lactating women.

Food Sources: The best natural sources are beef, lamb, pork, and chicken liver; deep-green leafy vegetables such as spinach, kale, and beet greens; asparagus, broccoli, wheat, bran, and yeast. It has been estimated that only 25 to 50 percent of the folic acid in food is biologically available. Cooking may reduce the folic content considerably. Sixty-eight percent of the folic acid is removed when wheat is processed into white flour.

OPTIMUM DAILY ALLOWANCE—ODA

For optimum general health, the basic Optimum Daily Allowance of folic acid is:

400–1200 mcg for men and women

In my clinical experience, I have found the following amounts of folic acid to be valuable for:

Cervical dysplasia . . . . 800 mcg three times a day
(under professional advice)

Folic acid anemia . . . . 800 mcg twice a day (higher
under professional advice)

Depression or anxiety . . . . . . 400–800 mcg

Remember: If you have a medical condition, or any psychiatric symptoms, please consult with your physician before taking supplements.

SUPPLEMENTS

Folic acid is available without a prescription in amounts up to 0.8 milligrams (800 micrograms) as an individual supplement or as part of a multivitamin formula. Stronger supplements are available only with a doctor's prescription.

TOXICITY AND ADVERSE EFFECTS

There is no known toxicity of folic acid. However, women who are taking folic acid supplements, especially if they are current or former users of oral contraceptives, are at risk for lower plasma zinc concentrations. I recommend that these women take additional zinc to prevent lowered zinc levels.

Chapter 17

PANTOTHENIC ACID

Our bodies convert pantothenic acid to coenzyme A, which is used in a variety of biological processes involving the metabolism of fats, carbohydrates, and protein, and the synthesis of steroids, cholesterol, bile, and hemoglobin. It is also needed for the production of two very important substances involved in nerve transmission, sphingosine and acetylcholine. Deficiencies in pantothenic acid have been shown to adversely affect the immune system in both humans and animals. Clearly, pantothenic acid is an essential nutrient. No RDA has been established; however, 4–7 milligrams per day are generally advised by professionals.

There are no documented cases of naturally occurring pantothenic acid deficiency. However, when deficiencies were artificially created in humans, headache, fatigue, insomnia, and nervous symptoms did occur. Some of these symptoms are no doubt due to the fact that pantothenic acid is vital for the healthy functioning of the adrenal gland. The adrenal gland connection is also why pantothenic acid has long been considered an "anti-stress" vitamin. Interestingly, laboratory animals fed a pantothenic-rich diet show significant improvement in exercise tolerance. This may hold true for humans too. Some studies actually show that pantothenic acid helps delay the onset of fatigue, especially when combined with other members of the B complex. One study in particular showed that human subjects given 10 milligrams of pantothenic acid daily were significantly better able to withstand cold water stress, which may be connected with its role in helping us resist stress in general.

There is some indication that pantothenic acid helps improve our ability to heal and withstand physical injury. For example, the surgical scars of supplemented laboratory animals healed better than the group that did not receive supplements. In another study, a preparation that included pantothenic acid reduced the effects of ultraviolet radiation on animals. Another preparation containing a pantothenic-like substance was applied to subjects with sports-related injuries; as a result, there was significant decrease in swelling and increase in joint mobility.

Some people with rheumatoid arthritis have significantly lower blood levels of pantothenic acid than normal people. In addition, the lower the levels of this nutrient, the more severe the symptoms may be. Studies have shown that when patients are given pantothenic acid, their symptoms of stiffness, disability, and pain are often alleviated; when the treatment is withdrawn, symptoms reappear.

Food Sources: Pantothenic acid appears in a wide variety of foods. The best sources are eggs, potatoes, salt water fish, pork, beef, milk, whole wheat, peas, beans, and fresh vegetables. Significant amounts of pantothenic acid are lost in foods when they are canned, cooked, frozen, or otherwise processed. For example, 50 percent of the pantothenic acid in grains is lost during the milling process.

OPTIMUM DAILY ALLOWANCE—ODA

For optimum general health, the basic Optimum Daily Allowance for pantothenic acid is:

25–300 mg for men and women

In my clinical experience, I have found the following amounts of pantothenic acid to be valuable for:

Joint inflammation . . . . 100–500 mg
Depression or anxiety . . . . 100–500 mg
Arthritis . . . . 50–500 mg

Remember: If you have a medical condition or psychiatric symptoms, please consult with your physician before taking supplements.

SUPPLEMENTS

Pantothenic acid appears in supplements as calcium pantothenate, which is 92 percent pantothenic acid and 8 percent calcium.

TOXICITY AND ADVERSE EFFECTS

Pantothenic acid has no known toxicity.

Chapter 18

BIOTIN

Biotin is an important coenzyme that is involved in the metabolism of carbohydrates and the synthesis of proteins and fats. It is not considered to be a true vitamin since it is made in our bodies by intestinal bacteria.

Biotin deficiency symptoms include a specific skin rash called seborrheic dermatitis (most commonly seen in infants) and hair loss; these conditions, when due to a deficiency, will respond to supplementation. However, I have never seen any convincing evidence to support the widely touted use of biotin as a cure for baldness. Biotin will work to restore hair only if there is an underlying skin condition due to a deficiency in this nutrient, which accompanies the hair loss.

Biotin deficiency has also been known to cause nausea, appetite loss, numbness, depression, and high blood cholesterol. There is some evidence that biotin supplementation helps prevent and treat nervous system disorders seen in patients undergoing chronic hemodialysis. Symptoms seen in these patients are similar to those seen in Alzheimer's disease: These include disorientation, speech disorders, memory failure, restless legs, tremors, and difficulty in walking.

There is no RDA for biotin. Only a few small groups of people have been found to be overtly biotin deficient. These groups are infants who are born with a genetic defect; people, such as bodybuilders, who eat large quantities of raw eggs; and those who are being treated with antibiotics or sulfa drugs for a long period of time (the drugs may reduce the synthesis of biotin by intestinal bacteria).

Food Sources: Foods high in biotin are chicken, lamb, pork, beef, veal, liver, yeast, soybeans, milk, cheese, salt water fish, whole wheat flour, and rice bran. Biotin is stable during normal cooking and processing. Eggs, another excellent source of biotin, contain a substance that inhibits biotin absorption in the body; however, cooking destroys this substance.

OPTIMUM DAILY ALLOWANCE—ODA

For optimum general health, the basic Optimum Daily Allowance for biotin is:

25–300 mcg for men and women

Remember: If you have a medical condition or psychiatric symptom, please consult with your physician before taking supplements.

SUPPLEMENTS

Biotin is available as d-biotin and is included in most B-complex and multivitamin supplements. It is also available as an individual supplement, but I have never felt the need to supplement biotin individually.

TOXICITY AND ADVERSE EFFECTS

Biotin is considered to be nontoxic.

Chapter 19

CHOLINE, INOSITOL, AND PABA

We do not know very much about these three nutrients, which are not considered essential vitamins because we are able to synthesize them in our bodies.

Both choline and inositol seem to be involved in the body's use of fats and cholesterol. Choline is needed for the transport and metabolism of fats. Inositol may be involved in the synthesis of phospholipids, which are essential to the digestion and absorption of fats, facilitate the uptake of fatty acids by the cells, and regulate the transport of material in and out of the cells. Both choline and inositol have been shown to alleviate or prevent the accumulation of abnormal quantities of fat in the liver.

Choline is also used by the body to make acetylcholine, a neurotransmitter in the brain. An adequate supply of this nutrient is critical for optimum nerve function. It has been demonstrated, for example, that a deficit of choline may play a role in the development of certain neurologic disorders such as Huntington's chorea, Parkinson's disease, and Alzheimer's disease.

Lecithin, a natural source of choline, has been used successfully to treat some cases of tardive dyskinesia, another neurological disorder. This condition, which results in facial twitches, is a common side effect of the heavy use of tranquilizers such as Thorazine. Lecithin has been widely advocated in the treatment of high serum cholesterol. However, studies have generally failed to prove its effectiveness.

PABA, which is short for para-aminobenzoic acid, seems to be needed for the formation of folic acid in the body and for the metabolism of protein. Although it has proved to be effective in combating gray hair in animals, I have never seen any evidence that this holds true for humans. PABA is a common ingredient in sunscreens because of its ability to protect against sunburn when applied to the skin. There is no evidence that oral doses of PABA have a similar effect.

There have been no known cases of naturally occurring choline, inositol, or PABA deficiency, and RDAs for these nutrients have not been established.

Food Sources: Choline is found in legumes, organ and muscle meats, milk, and whole-grain cereals and is particularly high in egg yolk. Inositol is distributed in fruits, vegetables, whole grains, meats, and milk. PABA is found in brewer's yeast, liver, kidney, whole grains, and molasses.

OPTIMUM DAILY ALLOWANCE—ODA

For optimum general health, the Optimum Daily Allowance is:

Choline: 25–300 mg for men and women
Inositol: 25–300 mg for men and women
PABA: 25–300 mg for men and women

There is not enough evidence at this time to warrant a high intake of these nutrients for most people, since large doses may even prove harmful if taken over an extended period of time.

However, if you are suffering from a neurological or neuromuscular disorder, you may want to try taking large amounts of lecithin under the advice of a professional. In my clinical practice, I have had good results using lecithin with mild cases of shingles—up to two capsules of 1200 mg each three times a day.

SUPPLEMENTS

Choline, inositol, and PABA are generally included in B-complex and multivitamin formulas, in similar amounts to the other B vitamins. They are also available as individual supplements.

Choline comes in three forms: choline bitartrate, choline dihydrogen citrate; and phosphatidyl choline (lecithin). I usually recommend lecithin, a natural substance high in this nutrient, since it is more absorbable and less irritating at higher levels than are the other two forms. Lecithin comes in several forms: capsules which contain oil, liquid lecithin, and granules.

Inositol is available in tablet and powder form. The tablets are preferable in that they are easier to take and cheaper than the powder. (It is said that the price of the powder is so high because it is allegedly purchased by those who intend to use it to cut cocaine. There is no evidence that inhalation of inositol confers any additional effects, or is of any therapeutic benefit.)

TOXICITY AND ADVERSE EFFECTS

There may be adverse effects if these nutrients are taken in high doses. Patients who have been treated with high oral doses of lecithin (choline) complain of dizziness, nausea, diarrhea, depression, and fishy odor. Recent studies show that high doses of PABA (8–48 grams daily) are associated with side effects such as malaise, fever, liver disease, and lowered white blood cell counts.

Chapter 20

VITAMIN C
(ASCORBIC ACID)

Ascorbic acid, or vitamin C as it is commonly called, has many functions in the body. Perhaps foremost is the major role it plays in the immune system, where the evidence is growing that it helps increase resistance to diseases including infections and cancer. For example, studies of animals and humans have shown that excesses of vitamin C stimulate the production of lymphocytes, an important component of our immune system. Ascorbic acid appears to be required by the thymus gland (one of the major glands involved in immunity) and increases the mobility of the phagocytes, the type of cell that "eats" harmful foreign invaders. Since vitamin C levels in the blood and body tissues decrease with age, it is not surprising that some elderly subjects who receive vitamin C supplements show enhanced immunity. Many laboratory studies have indicated that vitamin C inactivates a variety of viruses and bacteria in test tube conditions. Although the research that indicates that vitamin C can actually prevent colds is conflicting, many studies have shown that it can shorten the duration and lessen the intensity of the symptoms of upper respiratory infections. Taking vitamin C may not lessen the number of colds you get, but it will make them milder. Vitamin C has also been found to reduce the symptoms of asthma and allergies. I have had superb results using vitamin C in reducing these symptoms.

Another important role for vitamin C is the one it plays in our ability to handle all types of physical and mental stress. Vitamin C is needed by the adrenal glands to synthesize hormones, and the normally high levels of ascorbic acid in these glands are especially depleted during stress. Vitamin C levels are lowered by surgery and any kind of illness such as infections, wounds, and injuries; also by cigarette smoking and birth control pills. Research reveals that recovery from injury or surgery can be dramatically accelerated in individuals receiving vitamin C supplementation. In a study in which subjects were given eight to fifty times the RDA (460–3000 milligrams), recovery time was reduced by 50 to 70 percent; the higher the dosage, the shorter the recovery time.

Vitamin C is essential for the growth and repair of tissues in all parts of the body. It is needed for the formation of collagen (present in connective tissue), bone, and cartilage. Ascorbic acid is used in the repair of fractured bones. When given before and after dental extraction, it has been shown that the gum tissue heals more rapidly. It may reduce serum cholesterol in individuals with high cholesterol. It is needed to convert folic acid, a B vitamin, into its active form in our bodies. Vitamin C increases our ability to absorb iron from nonanimal foods such as raisins and spinach. It also plays a role in the storage of iron in the bone marrow, spleen, and liver. Vitamin C improves the bioavailability of selenium.

Vitamin C has also been shown to work as an antioxidant. (See Chapter 3.) It prevents other antioxidant vitamins such as A and E from becoming oxidized in the body, thus preventing the oxidation of our stored body fat. Its role as an antioxidant has implications for aging and the degenerative diseases that are associated with the aging process.

The studies of vitamin C for the treatment of cancer are, unfortunately, conflicting at this point. However, the case is far from closed. A pioneering study (in 1976, by Cameron and Pauling) of terminally ill cancer patients concluded that the patients who received supplemental ascorbic acid lived an average of 4.2 times longer than those who did not receive the supplement. Some supplemented patients lived 20 times longer. Subsequent studies have failed to duplicate these astounding results. However, laboratory studies have shown that ascorbic acid can inhibit the growth of leukemia cells and increase the cell-killing ability of various drugs and hormones. Since vitamin C appears to enhance chemotherapy in addition to boosting immunity, I and many other practitioners recommend vitamin C supplements to their patients who have cancer, usually in addition to conventional cancer therapy. Hospital protocol recommends that 500 milligrams of vitamin C be given to cancer patients.

Vitamin C's role in cancer prevention (as opposed to its treatment) is another story. Even traditionalists such as the National Cancer Institute and the American Cancer Society feel the evidence is strong enough to recommend a diet high in vitamin C as a possible preventive. Vitamin C's ability to enhance the immune system, discussed earlier, is just one way in which it contributes to cancer prevention. Another protective mechanism involves nitrosamines and similar substances. Nitrosamines are proved carcinogens in animals and humans. Our bodies are exposed to nitrosamines in food and cigarette smoke. In addition, we ingest nitrites and nitrates, the precursors of nitrosamines, in food (vegetables and cured packaged meats such as bacon, sausage, hot dogs, and ham), water, polluted air, and cigarette smoke. Our bodies make nitrosamines from these substances and many studies have shown that vitamin C blocks this process, and should therefore also block the formation of the tumors that nitrosamines could generate. Studies have correlated a high intake of dietary vitamin C with reduced risk of cancer of the stomach, colon, bladder, lung, esophagus, and cervix.

It is especially important that cigarette smokers take in adequate levels of vitamin C. For example, vitamin C has been found to be anti-carcinogenic in laboratory rodents who were exposed to benzopyrene. This is a very potent carcinogen found in cigarette smoke (including exhaled or "secondhand" smoke). Another study found that smokers needed a daily intake of nearly two and one-half times the RDA in order to maintain the same concentration of ascorbic acid in the body as nonsmokers.

Vitamin C acts in many ways to help prevent high blood pressure and atherosclerosis (hardening of the arteries which can lead to heart attacks and strokes). Both human and animal studies have linked increased levels of vitamin C with a reduction in serum cholesterol. Vitamin C may play a role in mobilizing cholesterol from the arteries to the liver, where it is converted into bile acids. It may help repair damaged arterial walls and so prevent cholesterol deposits from forming. In a clinical trial, patients with atherosclerosis given vitamin C could walk farther without feeling pain or breathlessness. In another study, surgical patients given 1000 milligrams of vitamin C daily had 50 percent lower incidence of deep vein thrombosis (a blood clot that can cut off the blood supply to a major organ such as the heart, lung, or brain). In humans, some studies have shown an increase in vitamin C is related to higher levels of high-density lipoproteins (HDLs). HDLs appear to protect you from heart disease.

The classical deficiency disease for vitamin C is scurvy. Early symptoms of scurvy are subtle and difficult to diagnose: lassitude, weakness, irritability, vague muscle and joint pains, and weight loss. Symptoms of advanced scurvy are bleeding gums, gingivitis, loosening of the teeth, and extreme weakness and fatigue. The RDA established to prevent these overt symptoms of scurvy is 60 milligrams for men and women.

Vitamin C clearly has many important uses, yet as a species, we humans are at high risk of not getting the amount we need. Unlike most other animals on this planet, we are incapable of producing vitamin C in our bodies. Neither can we store it for very long. Therefore, we must depend upon our food to supply us with what we need everyday. Many researchers argue that *optimum* intake of vitamin C is the amount that would be synthesized by humans if we had the enzyme necessary to make vitamin C. Animals which produce their own vitamin C have high levels of ascorbic acid in their tissues. It has been shown that mammals synthesize the equivalent of 3000–19,000 milligrams per day, when calculated for a human weighing 70 kilograms (154 pounds), dependent upon stress conditions. Maximum body pools (saturated tissue levels) in humans have been estimated at 1500 milligrams per day, but have been reevaluated by others at 5000 milligrams of vitamin C for a 70-kilogram person. It is estimated that a daily dose of about 200 milligrams of vitamin C would maintain a body pool of this size in a *healthy individual, totally devoid of stress of any kind.*

As another means of calculating the optimum daily intake, scientists have studied the handful of other animals that do not produce vitamin C: guinea pigs, primates, and certain fish. Their discovery also has startling implications for human beings: Per body weight, primates and guinea pigs eat the equivalent of 2000 milligrams of vitamin C per day; when under stress, they may eat the equivalent of up to 7000–10,000 milligrams of vitamin C per day. The recommended diet for guinea pigs and monkeys contains the equivalent of 1100 milligrams and 1250 milligrams daily. Others report that growth rate and other measures of good health indicate an optimum intake of the equivalent of 3500 milligrams. These data suggest that an optimum intake for humans may be 1000 milligrams or more daily. In still another study, it was determined that the typical caveman diet contained almost 400 milligrams of vitamin C daily.

And yet the RDA for ascorbic acid remains set at 60 milligrams!

Food Sources: The foods that are highest in vitamin C are broccoli, brussels sprouts, black currants, collards, guava, horseradish, kale, turnip greens, parsley, and sweet peppers. Also high on the list are cabbage, cauliflower, chives, kohlrabi, orange pulp, lemon pulp, mustard greens, beet greens, papaya, spinach, strawberries, and watercress. Medium sources are asparagus, lima beans, Swiss chard, gooseberries, red currants, grapefuit, limes, loganberries, melons, okra, tangerines, potatoes, and turnips. A newly discovered source very high in vitamin C is *terminalia ferdinandiana,* a member of the almond family with 2300–3150 milligrams per gram. (Notice that citrus fruits such as oranges and grapefruits do not have the highest ascorbic acid content; however, their skin is high in bioflavonoids, substances which increase the amount of vitamin C that is absorbed.)

Ascorbic acid is easily destroyed when exposed to oxygen; this process is accelerated by light and heat. Vegetables begin to lose vitamin C as soon as you cut them. Freshly squeezed oranges, which are not likely to be that high in vitamin C in the first place, quickly begin to lose their supply of this nutrient too. As a result, there is almost no vitamin C to speak of in juice sold in bottles or cartons. Since vitamin C is sensitive to heat and is lost when large quantities of water is used in cooking, vegetables should be eaten raw or lightly steamed or cooked in a small amount of water to retain the most of the vitamin.

OPTIMUM DAILY ALLOWANCE—ODA

For optimum general health, the basic Optimum Daily Allowance for vitamin C is:

500–5000 mg for men and women (along with 500–5000 mg bioflavonoids)

In my clinical experience, I have found the following amounts of vitamin C to be valuable for:

Surgery, wounds, injuries	5000–10,000 mg
High levels of stress	1000–5000 mg
Allergies or asthma	3000–7000 mg
Enhanced immunity	1000–5000 mg
Coronary heart disease prevention	500–3000 mg
Cancer prevention	5000–10,000 mg
Exposure to cigarette smoke and polluted air	1000–5000 mg
Bleeding gums	1000–3000 mg

Your optimum allowance varies depending upon the prevailing conditions. For example, you may want to raise your intake temporarily during times of stress, or if you have a cold or other form of infection. (Remember to decrease your supplementation *gradually* until it is back to your normal

ODA.) It is best if you spread your total intake of vitamin C over the course of the day. For example, if you take 3000 milligrams total, take 1000 milligrams at each meal. There are several advantages to this. Vitamin C is rapidly excreted from the body, and divided doses ensure a more constant level of blood and tissue saturation. It also reduces the likelihood of any adverse effects such as acid stomach or diarrhea.

Absorption varies widely from person to person. Studies have shown that one person may be able to absorb 3 grams of this vitamin without any excess spilling over into the urine; other subjects are only able to absorb 100 milligrams at one time, and will excrete anything over that.

Remember: If you have a medical condition, please consult with your physician before taking supplements.

SUPPLEMENTS

Vitamin C supplements are available both as ascorbic acid and mineral ascorbates. You should be aware that most vitamin C supplements contain vitamin C that has been synthesized from natural, inexpensive substances such as starch, molasses, or sago palm. The "natural" vitamin C found in supplements is extracted from rose hips, which contain 1 percent ascorbic acid. "Rose hips" vitamin C supplements contain mostly synthetic vitamin C; a vitamin C supplement made entirely from rose hips would be enormous in size and very expensive. However, rose hips may contain complementary substances (as yet undiscovered) that are useful along with the vitamin C, so there may be some advantage to taking this type. I recommend you buy ascorbic acid supplements which contain bioflavonoids (see page 110) because they have been shown to increase vitamin C absorption.

Ascorbic acid supplements are available mixed with minerals to form mineral ascorbates. The most readily available mineral ascorbate is calcium ascorbate, which is sometimes mixed with other mineral ascorbates such as magnesium ascorbate and sodium ascorbate. The advantage of calcium ascorbate is that it is a buffered form of vitamin C, a desirable trait for some individuals because it is nonacid and gentler to the stomach. More people can take higher oral doses of ascorbic acid in this form without getting acid stomach or diarrhea.

Vitamin C is widely available in tablet form. Some of these tablets are chewable; though convenient, they are not recommended for two reasons. First, chewable tablets are usually loaded with sugar. Second, they may cause the pH of the saliva to fall so low that calcium is leached from tooth enamel. Ascorbic acid is also available in powder form to be dissolved in liquids. The powder is cheaper, but less convenient to take; in addition, it can damage tooth enamel and so should be sipped through a straw if high dosages are taken frequently during the day.

TOXICITY AND ADVERSE EFFECTS

There is no proved toxicity for vitamin C. You may have heard vitamin C causes kidney stones, but there are no studies that show any relationship between vitamin C and the formation of kidney stones in *normal people.* However, if you have a history of kidney problems of any kind, you should take vitamin C only under the guidance of a qualified professional. With alterations in kidney function, the mechanism that handles vitamin C excretion may not be working properly so caution is warranted.

Early studies suggested that large doses of vitamin C destroy vitamin B-12 in the body; subsequent studies using improved techniques have shown that vitamin C does not have this effect.

However, one possible adverse side effect of very high levels of vitamin C is intestinal gas and looser stools. This effect is benign and completely reversible. In fact, many practitioners including myself advise using this effect as a guide in finding an individual's personal Optimum Daily Allowance.

In addition, another possible danger in taking very high doses of vitamin C—5000 milligrams a day and up—and then suddenly stopping the supplementation, is the risk of developing symptoms of "rebound scurvy." You can prevent this easily by reducing your dosage slowly over a period of a few weeks.

Vitamin C is used by the liver to detoxify drugs and other chemicals. It has been shown to prevent acetaminophen (aspirin substitutes such as Tylenol) toxicity to the liver without hindering the drug's effectiveness. However, with other long-acting drugs, you may want to consult with a professional about taking high doses of ascorbic acid.

BIOFLAVONOIDS

Bioflavonoids are now believed to be antioxidants. They are not quite vitamins, but they are present along with vitamin C in citrus fruit, in the white portion of the peel. Studies have shown that bioflavonoids ingested with vitamin C increase vitamin C absorption to a great extent. In addition, bioflavonoids strengthen capillary walls, preventing capillary damage which leads to bleeding disorders including spider veins, varicose veins, hemorrhages, and black and blue marks. They may enhance the ability of drugs to alleviate the symptoms of phlebitis. Bioflavonoids have been shown to have antibiotic-like activity. They may lower cholesterol. They were also shown to be potent anti-inflammatory agents and may prove useful for the treatment of arthritis. G. T. Terezhalmy of the National Naval Dental Center found that bioflavonoids together with vitamin C reduced the symptoms of oral herpes. In both human and animal research bioflavonoids were shown to have anticataract activity. Therefore, bioflavonoids may possibly be an effective treatment and prevention against cataracts.

OPTIMUM DAILY ALLOWANCE—ODA

For optimum general health, the Optimum Daily Allowance for bioflavonoids is:

500–5000 mg for men and women (to be taken along with an equivalent amount of vitamin C)

In my clinical experience, I have found the following amounts of bioflavonoids to be valuable for:

Inflamed joints	3000–10,000 mg
Capillary damage	500–5000 mg
Cataract prevention	1000–7000 mg
Herpes	1000–5000 mg

PART THREE
THE MINERALS

Chapter 21

CALCIUM

Our bodies contain approximately 1200 grams (about 2½ pounds) of calcium, 99 percent of which is stored in our bones and teeth. The remaining 1 percent of calcium (10–12 grams, or about one third of an ounce) is distributed throughout the body in the bloodstream and the fluids surrounding our cells.

Calcium is perhaps most well known for its role in the formation of the bones and tooth enamel. However, it also performs many other vital functions throughout our bodies. It is used to activate the enzymes involved in fat and protein digestion and in the production of energy. It is involved in blood clotting and the transmission of nerve impulses. Calcium regulates the contraction and relaxation of the muscles, including the heart. It aids in the absorption of many nutrients, especially vitamin B-12.

Recent studies indicate that low dietary intake of calcium may also be a factor in high blood pressure. Some scientists believe that the high incidence of hypertension in the United States may be a result of low calcium intake combined with high sodium intake. In one study, forty-eight hypertensive men were treated with 1000 milligrams of calcium for eight weeks. Twenty-one of them (44 percent) achieved a therapeutically meaningful reduction in their blood pressure. In many cases, the result was similar or superior to that achieved with blood pressure medication.

In another study, women with high blood pressure were given *either* 1500 milligrams of calcium or hypertensive medication for four years. The calcium-supplemented group achieved a significant drop in their systolic blood pressure; the unsupplemented group experienced a *rise* in their blood pressure, *even though they were taking hypertensive medication.* Studies have also revealed a correlation around the world between pregnancy-related hypertension and low calcium intake. In countries characterized by an average calcium intake of 1000 milligrams per day or more, pregnancy-related hypertension occurs in fewer than 1 out of 200 pregnancies; in societies where intake is under 500 milligrams per day, the incidence is ten to twenty times this.

Calcium supplementation is free of the unpleasant side effects so frequently encountered with antihypertensive drug treatment. These include impotence, fatigue, exercise intolerance and weight gain, dizziness, and impaired concentration. As the above studies indicate, calcium supplementation can be an effective nondrug means of preventing high blood pressure in high-risk individuals. In my experience, it can also be an effective, and perhaps a superior, nontoxic alternative to antihypertensive medication.

There is also some evidence that calcium may help prevent colon cancer. Epidemiological studies have shown that colon cancer incidence is lower in people who receive more sunlight exposure and consume more dairy foods. Some individuals prefer to get their milk in the form of yogurt since in addition to its calcium content it may protect in another way: yogurt supplies the "friendly" intestinal flora that inhibits the effects of known colonic carcinogens. A recent study suggested that individuals who eat a typical high-fat diet may be protected from colonic cancer by consuming 1200 milligrams of calcium daily. The authors found that within two to three months after supplementation was begun, tests of the subjects' colon linings showed that the number of fast-growing cells associated with cancer had significantly decreased.

However, most of the attention being paid to calcium is due to its role in maintaining strong, healthy bones. As we have seen, calcium exists not only in the bone, but performs various vital functions throughout the body. Our bones are designed to provide more than a rigid framework for our bodies; they also function as a kind of "bank" from which the body can draw the calcium it needs for other purposes. This is an ongoing, dynamic process during which bone, despite its seeming permanence, is a live tissue that is constantly being broken down (resorbed) and reformed. In the process, about 600–700 milligrams of calcium are exchanged in the bone of normal adults every day. Normally, if there is sufficient calcium being absorbed from the diet, the blood/bone calcium stays in balance and fluctuates only slightly. However, from the body's point of view, it is more important that there be enough calcium in the blood to keep the heart beating regularly, than it is to keep the bones strong and hard. So if the diet is deficient in calcium, the body will always choose to maintain a certain level of calcium in the blood by drawing it out of the bone. This is accomplished by a complex system involving hormones, especially parathyroid hormone and vitamin D. Even if there is adequate calcium in the diet, a lack of vitamin D will seriously impair the body's ability to make use of it.

This "survival mechanism" can cause some problems if a calcium-deficient diet is consumed over a long period of time. Eventually, there is so much calcium lost from the bone that osteoporosis (loss of bone mass or "shrinking" of the bone) occurs. The bones become porous, brittle, and so weak that a person may easily suffer a fracture from such normal activities as sneezing, bending over, or receiving a hug. The vertebrae of the spinal column may compress and/or fracture, causing pain, disability, loss of height, and a hunched-over appearance. If calcium is lost from the bones of the jaw, periodontal disease may result. This condition is occurring in epidemic proportions in an estimated 15 to 20 million Americans. Women over the age of fifty (postmenopausal) are especially at risk, but many younger people and older men are affected as well. Osteomalacia (softening of the bone) is another commonly seen problem that is due to inadequate calcium intake.

The growing consensus is that osteoporosis is not a disease that comes on suddenly in middle or old age. Many studies have correlated a long-term low-calcium diet, perhaps beginning at the age of thirty, perhaps earlier, with the development of osteoporosis and periodontal disease. In children, the deficiency symptom of inadequate calcium is rickets, a condition in which the bones grow too weak to support the weight of the child, with deformity as the highly visible result. There is some recent evidence that a suboptimum calcium intake in childhood may help set the stage for bone loss in later life, even though there were no obvious problems during childhood.

Unfortunately, because the body gives top priority to the maintenance of normal calcium levels in the blood, blood tests are an ineffective way to determine calcium levels in the bone, or in the diet. The blood may be perfectly normal, while the bone level is poor. The clinical signs of calcium depletion from the bone are insidious and not usually apparent until the symptoms of osteoporosis begin to appear. Even X rays are incapable of picking up bone loss until 30 to 40 percent of the bone has disappeared. Once osteoporosis is diagnosed, it can usually be slowed or halted with appropriate therapy, but it can be difficult to reverse. I feel the best course of action is prevention. That is why I recommend calcium supplementation be started as early as possible, and preferably by age twenty.

The RDA for calcium has been established at 800 milligrams (plus 400 milligrams for pregnant or lactating women). But new studies have indicated that this may not be enough for the entire population. Research has shown that a large percentage of patients with osteoporosis developed the condition even when their intake was at this level. The fact of the matter is, a person cannot develop osteoporosis and remain in calcium balance at the same time. If you consume calcium that is adequate for your particular set of circumstances, logic dictates that you will not develop osteoporosis.

Calcium intake is clearly a major factor in the development of osteoporosis, but it is not the only factor. There are many other life circumstances that influence the absorption and utilization of the amount of calcium we do take in. These include other elements in the diet, the amount of exercise we get, and any medication taken.

How much phosphorus we take in influences our requirement for calcium. Most researchers advise that the ratio of calcium to phosphorus should be at least 1:1. In other words, that we should take in at least as much calcium as we do of phosphorus. If phosphorus is much higher, it may impair the absorption of calcium, as well as increase the amount drawn out of the bone. If our diet contains many phosphorus-rich foods such as meats, soft drinks, and food additives, our phosphorus intake may be too high to maintain a good calcium balance.

Studies have also linked high-protein diets and high-fat diets, particularly in foods of animal origin, with the loss of calcium from the bone. However, it is difficult to isolate other factors such as vitamin D, calcium, and phosphorus intake in these studies. Therefore, the results have been conflicting.

A recent study suggests that an adequate amount of *all* the micronutrients can make a significant difference in the body's proper and efficient metabolism of calcium. One group of women was given a calcium and vitamin D supplement; they experienced an improvement in bone density. The other group received a balanced supplement of calcium, vitamin D, plus 100 percent of the RDA for over fifteen other vitamins and minerals. This group experienced a *two to three times* greater increase in bone density.

Many scientists agree the RDA for calcium should be raised to at least 1000–1500 milligrams, particularly for women. Interestingly enough, recent research has discovered that our ancient human ancestors who lived during the Paleolithic Era ingested approximately 1600 milligrams of calcium per day. Evolutionary theory suggests that we are genetically "programmed" to require a similar amount. The richest food source is milk and dairy products. Three glasses of milk or their equivalent are needed to attain the RDA of 800 milligrams, but many people do not include anywhere near this amount in their diets. While the lactose in milk may increase calcium absorption, we are not sure whether lactose-intolerant people (who have trouble digesting milk) experience an impairment in calcium absorption. They are likely, however, to avoid milk products, and so are at particularly high risk of calcium deficiency for this reason.

One study has found that two thirds of the women in America between the ages of eighteen and thirty (the age at which peak bone mass is developing) ingest less than the RDA. After the age of thirty-six, three quarters have calcium intakes less than the RDA. Fully one fourth of all U.S. women ingest less than 300 milligrams on any given day. Further exacerbating the situation is that absorption of whatever calcium is in the diet begins to decrease during the ages of forty to fifty; and in some perhaps as early as thirty. After menopause, estrogen levels decrease, an event which has also been implicated in bone loss. Estrogen therapy, which may have some disturbing side effects, is often prescribed in an attempt to prevent bone loss in postmenopausal women. However, in addition to normal dietary calcium, an increase in calcium intake of about 500 milligrams per day is required to produce the same balance effect as moderate doses of estrogen. Therefore many scientists prefer calcium supplements over the hormone therapy. I certainly do.

I also advise my patients to get regular physical exercise because studies have shown that physical exercise may improve calcium absorption and utilization. It may therefore play a crucial role in the prevention and/ or treatment of osteoporosis. Exercise has been shown to increase bone mass in athletes, in the elderly, and in people recovering from the decrease in bone mass that occurs during a decrease in physical activity. Loss of bone mass is most pronounced in people undergoing full bed rest, who lose 200–300 milligrams calcium per day. A diet that is adequate for a healthy adult may not provide enough calcium to offset prior illness-related losses. Increasing the calcium intake alone during the illness will not offset these losses either. However, resumed physical activity combined with adequate calcium intake will restore the bone.

Food Sources: Dairy foods such as milk, cheese, and yogurt are outstanding sources of calcium. If we do not consume such foods, it is extremely difficult to achieve a satisfactory intake of calcium from foods. In addition to its being a superb source of calcium, milk contains lactose, a substance that may increase the absorption of calcium in our bodies. Other sources which can make a substantial contribution include canned salmon and sardines (including the bones) and green leafy vegetables such as collard greens, turnip greens, and mustard greens. Clams, oysters, and shrimp are also good sources of calcium, followed by kale, broccoli, soybeans, and soybean products such as tofu.

It has been estimated that we actually absorb as little as 20 to 40 percent of the calcium in our food. Part of the problem may be oxalic acid, a substance found in spinach, Swiss chard, beet greens, cocoa, and rhubarb, which may bind with calcium to prevent its absorption in the colon. Phytic acid, or phytates, a substance found in the outer layers of cereal grains, may also interfere with calcium absorption. However, the evidence is inconclusive and many scientists discount it. This effect appears to occur only when the calcium intake is low and the oxalic acid or phytate intake is quite high. In addition, the fermentation of yeast, as found in leavened bread, destroys much of the phytate in the flour. In fact, when vegetarians were studied, it was found that they have less incidence of osteoporosis than nonvegetarians. Since vegetarians as a group eat a diet high in phytates, it seems unlikely that calcium absorption is significantly affected.

OPTIMUM DAILY ALLOWANCE—ODA

For optimum general health, the basic Optimum Daily Allowance for calcium is:

1000–1500 mg for men and women

In my clinical experience, I have found the following amounts of calcium to be valuable for:

Osteoporosis	1200–2000 mg
High blood pressure	1000–1500 mg
Broken bones and fractures	1000–2000 mg

Calcium should be taken with magnesium in a ratio of 2:1, and with vitamin D to aid in absorption. Since the body is unable to absorb 1000 milligrams all at once, divide your total ODA into halves or thirds and take them two or three times a day.

Remember: If you have a medical condition, please consult with your physician before taking supplements.

SUPPLEMENTS

Calcium supplements are available as tablets, as flavored chewable squares, and in liquid form. The supplements generally combine pure or "elemental" calcium with other chemicals or "salts." The most available forms are calcium carbonate, calcium lactate, and calcium gluconate. When buying calcium supplements, remember to consider the amount of elemental calcium, not the amount of calcium salts. Of the three forms, calcium carbonate contains the greatest amount of elemental calcium (40 percent). Many people prefer this form because the higher calcium content means they need to take fewer pills to obtain their Optimum Daily Requirement. Another factor to consider is absorbability. I generally recommend calcium carbonate and calcium lactate since they appear to be very absorbable. Calcium citrate has recently been shown to be the most absorbable, particularly in the elderly. However, this form is rather costly.

I advise you to take your calcium supplements along with magnesium and vitamin D because they all work together to enhance each others' absorption and utilization in the body. The calcium-to-magnesium ratio should be approximately 2:1. Fortunately, there are now many supplements that contain calcium carbonate or calcium lactate and magnesium in the proper proportions. There are also supplements that combine calcium with vitamin D.

Dolomite is a supplement that contains both calcium and magnesium; however, this product is the least absorbable, and I do not recommend it as a supplement. Bone meal, another source of calcium, is highly absorbable. However, this form contains substantial amounts of phosphorus and most people get quite enough (and often too much) phosphorus from their diets.

Many antacids are being promoted as calcium supplements since these products contain calcium carbonate. However, most contain aluminum, a mineral that can have many deleterious effects on the body. One study showed that these adverse effects include high levels of calcium excreted in the urine, bone resorption (loss of minerals from the bone), impaired fluoride absorption, and phosphorus depletion, all of which may ironically contribute to bone disease.

TOXICITY AND ADVERSE EFFECTS

There are no known toxic effects for calcium. An FDA panel concluded that calcium intakes of 1000–2500 milligrams daily do not result in hypercalcemia (high levels of calcium in the blood). Hypercalcemia may be seen in certain medical conditions and when there is an overdose of vitamin D, but a high intake of calcium is not in itself a causative factor. Development of kidney stones in connection with high calcium intake is rare.

Some people report a feeling of relaxation and drowsiness after taking calcium supplements. This has never been documented in a scientific study. However, if you notice this particular effect, you can do what I suggest to my patients: namely, offset (and perhaps take advantage) of this effect by taking your supplements in the evening before retiring.

Chapter 22

PHOSPHORUS

Phosphorus is the second most abundant mineral in the body after calcium. There are approximately 600–700 grams (1 1/4–1 1/2 pounds) in the average-sized person, or about 1 percent of the total weight. As is the case with calcium, most of the body's phosphorus (80–90 percent) is in the bone and teeth. The rest is distributed throughout the body in the cells, blood, and other fluids. The ratio of calcium to phosphorus in the bone is about 2:1; however, we have a much higher proportion of phosphorus in the soft tissues.

In addition to its contribution to the hardness of the bones which support our bodies, phosphorus plays a part in almost every important chemical reaction in the body. Most of its action has to do with the utilization of fats, protein, and carbohydrates. One function is to combine with fats in the blood to become phospholipids. Phospholipids in turn become part of the cell structure that is responsible for regulating the transport of materials in and out of the cell. Phosphorus is also involved in the transport of fats in the circulatory system.

Phosphorus is involved in a variety of processes which store and produce energy. For example, it is part of such cellular processes as muscle contraction, the transfer of nerve impulses, hormone secretion, and protein synthesis. It is also a component of nucleic acids (DNA and RNA), which control heredity and the replication of cells. Many of the B vitamins are effective only when combined with this mineral in the body. Finally, phosphorus is involved in our buffer system, which keeps the body pH in balance.

Phosphorus is obviously essential to our good health. Fortunately, most people have no trouble getting more than the Recommended Daily Allowance of 800 milligrams from their food. Although there is some evidence that phytates in food interfere with the absorption of essential minerals, there is some doubt whether this occurs on a scale that is of practical importance. Long-term phytate consumption has not been specifically investigated. However, vegetarians, who consume a high-fiber diet rich in phytates, have not been shown to be deficient in phosphorus. Long-term use of aluminum-containing antacids, however, may deplete the body of phosphorus to such a degree that deficiency is a real possibility. Symptoms of phosphorus deficiency are weakness, loss of appetite, loss of bone mass, and loss of calcium.

In general, phosphorus is one of the few micronutrients of which we are far more likely to have too much than too little. It is suggested that phosphorus and calcium intake should be approximately equal (1:1), even though the ratio in bone is 2:1. The average daily intake is between 1500 and 1600 milligrams. This means that in most diets, the phosphorus intake exceeds the calcium intake, and this may be in part responsible for creating calcium loss.

The actual absorption, storage, and excretion of phosphorus is dependent on mechanisms involving vitamin D and parathyroid hormone. Like calcium, phosphorus exists in a complex give-and-take relationship between the bones, the blood, and the soft tissues of the body. It is continuously being deposited and released from the bone "bank" as the blood levels fluctuate in response to dietary intake and excretion. In addition, phosphorus levels and calcium levels influence each other. Excess phosphorus consumption is common. There is a convincing body of evidence suggesting that a diet overly rich in phosphorus, along with long-term low calcium intakes and high protein intake, is a major dietary factor in the demineralization of the bone which leads to osteoporosis. (See Chapter 21, "Calcium" for more information on calcium and osteoporosis.)

Food Sources: Phosphorus is found in nearly all foods, but is especially high in carbonated soft drinks, milk and dairy products, meat, and fish. Nuts, beans, and grains are also high in phosphorus.

OPTIMUM DAILY ALLOWANCE—ODA

For optimum general health, the Optimum Daily Allowance for most people can usually be met through dietary sources. Possible exceptions may include the elderly, menopausal women, and individuals on restricted diets. For this population, the ODAs are:

200–400 mg for men and women

Remember: If you have a medical condition, please consult with your physician before taking supplements.

SUPPLEMENTS

Rather than supplementing phosphorus, most people appear to require a *reduction* of phosphorus in their diets. Particularly high-phosphorus foods to watch out for include meat and carbonated beverages. Traditionally, a calcium-to-phosphorus ratio of 1:1 is recommended. However, as a general rule, a higher percentage of phosphorus is absorbed from the diet (70 percent) than of calcium (40 percent). In addition, the calcium-to-phosphorus ratio in the bone is 2:1. Bearing this in mind, you may want to manipulate the ratio slightly in favor of calcium in order to maintain a more favorable balance in the body.

TOXICITY AND ADVERSE EFFECTS

Too much phosphorus may lead to an increase in the excretion of calcium, and consequently to osteoporosis.

Chapter 23

MAGNESIUM

Our bodies contain between 20 and 28 grams of magnesium, approximately half of which is found in the bone. Along with calcium and phosphorus, sufficient magnesium is required for strong, healthy bones.

The rest of the body's magnesium is a part of many enzyme systems that are involved in the flow of certain elements across the cell membranes. One of magnesium's most important roles is that of maintaining the function of the nerves. It is also used in muscle relaxation. When calcium flows into muscle tissue cells, the muscle contracts. When calcium leaves and magnesium replaces it, the muscle relaxes. These functions are no doubt related to the association of magnesium deficiency with the occurrence of muscle spasms, tremors, and convulsions.

Low magnesium may also be associated with psychiatric problems. In a study of 165 boys, it was found that those with symptoms of depression, schizophrenia, and sleep disturbances had lower levels of magnesium in the blood. In another study, it was found that the average magnesium levels of autistic children were also well below average. In fact, there is some evidence that autistic children may improve when given large doses of magnesium along with vitamin B-6. In adults, insufficient magnesium may be accompanied by a loss of sensation in the extremities and, if severe, tremors, convulsions, muscle contractions, confusion, delirium, and behavioral disturbances. One study found that psychiatric patients who had attempted suicide had lower magnesium levels than either nonsuicidal psychiatric patients or healthy individuals.

Magnesium also works with the enzymes in the body to break down sugar stored in the liver to create energy. These reactions are essential whenever energy is expended.

Magnesium interacts with other substances known to affect the muscle tone of the blood vessels, such as sodium, potassium, and calcium. This may be why so many studies suggest that inadequate magnesium may play an important role in the development and progression of diseases of the blood vessels. For example, there is evidence that magnesium supplementation is effective in lowering some types of high blood pressure in individuals with low magnesium levels. In addition, studies have shown that people suffering from angina, which can be caused by a spasm of the blood vessel leading to the heart, are helped by magnesium supplementation. People with high blood pressure often experience spasms in the blood vessels of the retina. As a result, there may be some damage which can eventually affect their vision. People suffering from this condition tend to have low levels of magnesium, and treatment with magnesium supplements has been shown to cause the disease to regress. Diabetes is another disease that damages the blood vessels of the retina, and this can lead to severe vision problems and even blindness. There is evidence that low levels of magnesium may be an additional risk factor in the development and progression of this complication.

Magnesium may prove useful in preventing certain pregnancy complications such as prematurity and intrauterine growth retardation.

Since magnesium is so widely distributed in foods, severe deficiencies are most often recognized in those whose food intake is low or imbalanced such as alcoholics and diabetics. However, many other groups of people may be at risk. Those undergoing diuretic therapy or treatment with the drug cyclosporin A also may have depleted magnesium. In addition, magnesium may be too low in people with malabsorption syndromes or gastrointestinal disease such as Crohn's disease. We are also beginning to recognize that bulimics are at risk because of their prolonged diarrhea and/or vomiting. Oral contraceptive use has been found to lower blood magnesium. Since low magnesium results in blood clots, this may be at least part of the answer to the question of why there is a higher incidence of thrombosis among women on the Pill. Stress has also been implicated in depleted magnesium levels, which may account for the typical "Type A" personality's possible increased risk for cardiovascular disease. One study suggests that stress may also be in part responsible for the lowered magnesium levels in women with premenstrual tension.

The RDA for magnesium is 350 milligrams per day for men; 300 milligrams per day for women, plus 150 milligrams if pregnant or lactating.

Food Sources: Magnesium is widely distributed in foods. Those with the highest content of this mineral are milk and dairy products, meat, fish and seafood, nuts, blackstrap molasses, soybeans, peanuts, seeds, and wheat germ. Whole grains such as oatmeal, cornmeal, and rice are good sources.

Bear in mind, however, that the magnesium content of food varies considerably with the magnesium content of the soil in which the food is grown. In addition, much of the magnesium in food is lost during processing. For example, milling removes 59 percent of the magnesium from whole wheat. Cooking foods in water also leaches out this mineral.

OPTIMUM DAILY ALLOWANCE—ODA

For optimum general health, the basic Optimum Daily Allowance for magnesium is:

500–750 mg for men and women

In my clinical experience, I have found the following amounts of magnesium to be valuable for:

Osteoporosis . . . .   500–1000 mg
High blood pressure . . . .   500–750 mg
Oral contraceptive use . . . . .   500–750 mg
Angina . . . .   500–1000 mg (under professional supervision)

Remember: If you have a medical condition, please consult your physician before taking supplements.

SUPPLEMENTS

I recommend magnesium supplements as magnesium carbonate or magnesium oxide. Magnesium oxide contains the most pure magnesium (60 percent); equally common is magnesium carbonate (40 percent magnesium). Chelated magnesium (bound to amino acids) is also available. As with calcium supplements, the potency is determined by the elemental magnesium content. Magnesium sulfate is commonly known as epsom salt.

Magnesium works together with calcium and phosphorus, and so must be in balance in the body. Therefore both calcium and magnesium supplements should be taken. (Food usually supplies enough phosphorus.)

The consensus is that the calcium-to-magnesium ratio should be about 2:1, and that is what I usually recommend. There are supplements available which contain both calcium and magnesium in the 2:1 ratio (see Chapter 21, "Calcium"). Some researchers believe the ratio should be closer to 1:1; however, studies suppporting this ratio are lacking at this time. Many people compromise and take in a ratio of 2:1½.

TOXICITY AND ADVERSE EFFECTS

Toxicity is rare, except in individuals with kidney failure. Large amounts of magnesium salts (3000–5000 milligrams daily) have a cathartic effect and magnesium-containing products are often used as over-the-counter laxatives. These products, which include Epsom salts, milk of magnesia, and magnesium citrate, work by drawing fluid into the intestines, thereby stimulating contractions. Toxicity symptoms have been noted in subjects who were treated with 9000 milligrams.

Chapter 24

ZINC

Our bodies contain approximately 2–3 grams of zinc, which is distributed throughout the body. Zinc is an essential component of over twenty enzymes associated with many different metabolic processes. The highest concentrations of zinc are found in the eyes, liver, bone, prostate, semen, and hair.

However, there are no true storage depots for this mineral. Although relatively large amounts are found in the bone along with other minerals, it does not appear that this zinc is readily available to the body. We are dependent upon a continual external supply, as the relatively small body pool of biologically available zinc appears to be used rather rapidly. Therefore, deficiency signs tend to appear quite soon after depletion. It is now recognized that the following may indicate subclinical zinc deficiency: impaired ability to heal, impaired acuity of taste and smell, loss of appetite, and impaired night vision. Prolonged zinc deficiency may result in failure to grow, mental disturbances, lethargy, skin changes, and susceptibility to frequent infections. Testicular function may also be adversely affected. Since oysters are quite high in zinc, this is probably the origin of the oyster's reputation as an aphrodisiac.

Perhaps the most critical role zinc plays is in the synthesis of the nucleic acids RNA and DNA, which are essential for cell division, cell repair, and cell growth. This would help explain its involvement in growth and development and in aiding reproductive function. There is evidence that the importance of zinc for growth begins as early as in the womb. Several studies link low zinc levels with complications during pregnancy, miscarriage, and birth defects. Studies have also found large percentages of apparently healthy children to be deficient in zinc. They showed symptoms of suboptimal growth, in addition to a loss of taste acuity and poor appetite. When their zinc intake was increased, these symptoms improved. Animal and human studies in children and adults suggest that lethargy, passivity, and apathy are symptoms of marginal zinc deficiency since these behavioral problems have improved with zinc supplementation.

Other studies support zinc as a factor in wound healing. When hospital patients who were marginally deficient in zinc were given extra zinc, it helped restore the rate of healing to normal. Zinc may therefore be of benefit to people who have undergone surgery, broken bones, and wounds. Some physicians are starting to prescribe zinc to stimulate the healing process.

There is some evidence that zinc levels fall after physical and mental stress. It has been discovered, for example, that zinc is depleted during upper respiratory infection accompanied by fever. In addition, severe burn victims have only two thirds the normal amount of zinc in their blood. Strenuous exercise has been shown to lead to significant losses of zinc, probably due to the increase in glucose metabolism, which requires zinc.

Zinc is important in body systems that undergo a rapid turnover of cells. This includes the gastrointestinal system, and particularly the taste buds. This may explain why in early zinc deficiency there is a change in the ability to taste foods. This may be accompanied by similar changes in the ability to smell. Foods may either have no taste or smell at all, or they may taste or smell unpleasant. All these factors contribute to a loss of appetite, but may be so insidious that they go unnoticed. Many of my elderly patients report a heightened sense of taste after a few weeks of zinc supplementation. They find this development quite remarkable, since they didn't realize they had lost taste sensitivity before the supplementation.

Zinc may play a multifaceted role in protecting us from harmful substances. It protects the liver from damage due to poisoning from the common cleaning solvent carbon tetrachloride. Zinc is known to prevent the absorption of lead and cadmium and so may alleviate the toxic effects of these heavy metals which may be present in drinking water. Lead exposure can occur due to water flowing through lead plumbing, air pollution, car and bus exhaust fumes, and industrial waste. Cadmium, which can be leached from galvanized or black polyethylene pipes, is also present in exhaust fumes and industrial waste, and has been shown to raise blood pressure. Zinc may also be protective against the harmful effects of free radicals through its influence on cell membrane stability.

Zinc may also exert a protective influence by boosting the immune system. Many studies have shown that a zinc deficiency can impair a large variety of immune functions and defense mechanisms in animals. Some studies have shown similar effects in humans. These effects include abnormalities and eventual shrinking of the spleen, thymus, and lymph nodes; depression in the number and activity of killer cells; and impaired antibody production. These conditions were correctable with zinc supplementation. Low zinc levels, often accompanied by high copper levels, have been reported in people with many types of cancer. In a 1981 study, it was found that people with a certain type of lung cancer survived a significantly longer time if they had high levels of zinc in their blood. Since the beneficial effects of zinc on immunity are so well documented, and the therapy is nontoxic and inexpensive, some researchers suggest further studies involving immune deficiency diseases. Many of my patients who get frequent colds and sore throats have shown a marked decrease in these outbreaks after using zinc supplements.

Many studies suggest that there is a relationship between zinc depletion and anorexia nervosa. Researchers theorize that inadequate zinc might somehow initially help trigger the development of this disease, which then depletes zinc levels further, worsening the disease symptoms, and so on, in a vicious cycle. My patients, and those of other practitioners, who suffer from this condition have improved after zinc supplementation, which leads me to believe it may play a role in the treatment, and perhaps the prevention, of this serious disease.

The highest concentration of zinc in the human body is in the eye, especially the iris and retina. Although the exact mechanism of its functions are largely unknown, zinc seems to be involved with the activation of vitamin A in the eye and thus is a factor in night vision. There is a growing body of evidence to indicate that zinc is also related to other eye conditions such as impaired color discrimination, cataract formation, and optic neuritis (inflammation of the optic nerve).

The RDA for zinc is 15 milligrams per day for adults; 20 milligrams for pregnant women, and 25 milligrams for lactating women. In spite of its importance and seemingly wide availability in food, evidence indicates that many people do not get enough zinc from their diets. Marginally low intakes are common in large areas of the country because the soil is deficient in this mineral. (In fact, many farm animals were found to be deficient and now eat feed that has been enriched with zinc.) A 1979 study detected an average intake of 8.6 milligrams per day for humans, or just over half the RDA. In another survey, the zinc intake of elderly people was on the average less than one half the RDA, indicating this group is particularly at risk. It is worthwhile noting that the people in this survey suffered from the loss in the ability to taste that is so common among this age group. In another study of the elderly, it was found that senile purpura (purple spots under the skin caused by bleeding) may be due to a zinc deficiency.

People with a hereditary disease called acrodermatitis enteropathica are not able to absorb zinc. Those with other malabsorption syndromes such as Crohn's disease, celiac disease, and short bowel syndrome are at risk for inadequate zinc, as are people with chronic kidney disease, sickle cell disease, cystic fibrosis, pancreatic insufficiency, and other chronically debilitating diseases. These individuals may have subtle signs of zinc deficiency including loss of appetite, impaired night vision, and depressed immune and mental functions. In one study, patients with highly active Crohn's disease had only 60 percent of the normal zinc level in the blood.

Several drugs can interfere with zinc absorption and metabolism. These include such commonly used substances as alcohol, steroids, oral contraceptives, and diuretics. The hormones in the Pill are the probable cause for the dip in zinc levels; zinc levels are also lower during pregnancy. Oral contraceptives have been found to reduce folic acid levels in some women, and in these cases folic acid supplements may be advised. However, folic acid in large doses has been reported to lower zinc concentrations in the blood, so these women may be particularly prone to develop a zinc deficiency and I feel should take supplements accordingly.

Some research on the use of diuretics for hypertension suggests that there may be many possible links between zinc depletion and unexplained side effects of these drugs. Impotency, for example, may be connected to low zinc levels, and not to the drugs themselves. Diuretic therapy and the resulting losses of zinc before or after myocardial infarction (heart attack) have important implications because this may retard the healing of the injured heart.

Zinc has been shown to inhibit the production of prolactin, a pituitary hormone. According to a recent study, men with kidney disease undergoing dialysis showed lower levels of zinc and high levels of prolactin. The lowered zinc may be the cause of the elevated prolactin, which can lead to such distressing effects as the secretion of breast milk, enlarged breasts, and sexual dysfunction.

The water you drink may affect zinc levels. Excessive copper, a common source of which is copper pipes, worsens an already existing zinc deficiency. In addition, there is some evidence that the calcium bicarbonate in hard tap water may interfere with zinc absorption and utilization.

Food Sources: Some zinc is found in nearly all foods, but is especially plentiful in meats, poultry (particularly dark meat), fish, seafood (oysters are notably high), liver, eggs, legumes such as peanuts, and whole grains. Approximately 73 percent of the zinc is removed from whole grains during the milling process that produces white flour. The flour is then "enriched," which replaces several vitamins and iron, but not zinc.

The biological availability of zinc in different foods varies; it is estimated that as little as 40 percent of dietary zinc is actually absorbed. Some studies have suggested that the zinc in animal meats and seafood is better absorbed than the zinc in vegetable foods. Zinc deficiency is known to occur in populations whose zinc intake is far in excess of the RDA, but is derived solely from vegetable (cereal) sources. This has led to the concern that vegetarians may need a higher intake of zinc. However, when vegetarians were recently studied, it was found that they have adequate zinc levels. It may be that the soybean products popular in vegetarian cuisine are a factor in supplying the extra zinc and in enhancing its absorption.

OPTIMUM DAILY ALLOWANCE—ODA

For optimum general health, the basic Optimum Daily Allowance for zinc is:

22.5–50 mg for men and women

In my clinical experience, I have found the following amounts of zinc to be valuable for:

Decreased sense of taste and smell . . . . 30–50 mg
Poor night vision . . . . 30–50 mg
Enhanced wound healing . . . . 30–50 mg
Enhanced immunity . . . . 30–50 mg
Prostatitis . . . . 30–100 mg

Remember: If you have a medical condition, please consult with your physician before taking supplements.

SUPPLEMENTS

Zinc is available as individual supplements, or as part of many multivitamin and multimineral formulas. In supplements, pure or "elemental" zinc is combined with other chemicals. Of these, I feel zinc gluconate, sometimes referred to as chelated zinc, is the best choice for most people. Zinc sulphate is the least expensive, but it can be very irritating to the stomach. Many practitioners feel that zinc piccolinate is the most absorbable form; however it is very expensive and so I usually reserve it for my patients who have poor absorption. Zinc orotate, another expensive form of zinc, is also promoted as the most absorbable form, but thus far this has not been proven.

Since zinc supplements combine elemental or pure zinc with another chemical, when buying supplements you must consider the amount of elemental zinc; the zinc equivalent is commonly listed on the product label. For example, 80 milligrams of zinc gluconate usually contains 10 milligrams of elemental zinc; 220 milligrams of zinc sulfate supplies 50 milligrams of elemental zinc.

TOXICITY AND ADVERSE EFFECTS

The symptoms of zinc toxicity are gastrointestinal irritation and vomiting. Zinc is actually recognized as an emetic (vomit inducer). However, this form of toxicity only occurs when 2000 milligrams or more have been ingested. Studies have shown that even when up to ten times the RDA (150 milligrams) of zinc is given for prolonged periods of time, there are no adverse reactions.

There is some evidence that excessive intake of zinc may lower copper and aggravate a marginal copper deficiency. This may in fact be a beneficial, rather than an adverse, effect for many people. Although copper is an essential nutrient, a large number of people have copper levels that are far too high for optimum health, so this study offers an intriguing new possible use for zinc. However, this matter is still unresolved, and some researchers recommend that patients on long-term zinc supplementation have their copper levels monitored.

Short-term experiments suggest that 150 milligrams of zinc twice a day decrease HDL cholesterol and raise LDL and/or serum cholesterol, causing a less desirable ratio. However, studies are needed to assess long-term effects. The results of another study, using 50 milligrams of zinc per day, showed the opposite effect: HDL cholesterol increased and overall cholesterol decreased. In addition, diastolic blood pressure decreased. At one time, my HDLs were 46 and my total cholesterol was 225. After three years of taking 100 milligrams of zinc daily, my HDLs are 98 and my cholesterol is 185. My HDL levels certainly have not suffered by taking excess zinc. Of course, I take a *balance* of other supplements along with zinc, as well as do aerobic exercise three times a week.

Chapter 25

IRON

Iron is found in all of our cells. Approximately 75 percent of it is in the hemoglobin of our red blood cells, which is responsible for carrying oxygen from our lungs to all the parts of the body. Hemoglobin also indirectly aids in the return of carbon dioxide to the lungs. About 5 percent of our iron is found in myoglobin, an iron protein complex that is found in the muscles and which supplies extra energy when needed. Iron is also present in many enzymes which are involved in the production of energy.

The major deficiency disease for iron is hypochromic microcytic anemia. In this form of anemia, the red blood cells are pale in color and smaller than normal. They have low amounts of hemoglobin, and as a result, the tissues of the body become oxygen-starved. The symptoms of iron deficiency anemia are listlessness, fatigue, irritability, difficulty swallowing, paleness, heart palpitations during exertion, and a general lack of well-being.

However, the symptoms of anemia appear only after all the body stores of iron have been depleted. Therefore, the usual tests for anemia are an unsatisfactory means of determining the presence of iron depletion. Even in the absence of anemia, iron deficiency may have a detrimental effect on behavior and learning ability. For example, chronically fatigued women, whose tests nevertheless indicated they were nonanemic, were studied. The researchers concluded that some of these women might have been suffering from iron deficiency even though their hemoglobin was in the accepted range. Apparently, their normal range for hemoglobin was higher than average. When college students were studied, it was found that low iron may play a part in faulty attention span. Another study indicated that iron supplementation in iron-deficient children improved their ability to learn. In infants, studies have revealed similar findings: Both those with anemia and those with signs of deficiency (but no anemia) showed significant improvement in mental development scores when supplemented with iron.

Iron is also of key importance in maintaining many of the healthy functions of our immune system and our defenses against disease. Either too much or too little may create problems; however, most problems are due to a deficiency. These include increased susceptibility to infection, reduced white blood cell counts, and impaired antibody production.

Other widely diverse signs of possible iron deficiency have recently come to light. Angular cheilosis, an inflammation of the corners of the mouth, has most frequently been seen in vitamin B deficiencies. However, according to one report, iron deficiency was present in a much higher percentage of sufferers of this condition. Animal experiments suggest that iron deficiency may contribute to high fat levels in the blood and liver. In addition, new data indicate that a craving for salt may be a sign of iron deficiency.

Of all the nutrients, the iron allowance is the most difficult to provide. This is why iron deficiency is the most common single nutrient deficiency in the world. Vast numbers of individuals become deficient in iron at some time in their lives, and large segments of the population are chronically deficient. Iron deficiency is far from uncommon in men, children, and in the elderly. It is my experience that most men and women require iron supplementation.

However, the highest risk category is menstruating women. Healthy men have an iron reserve in the body of 1000 milligrams and lose an average of 1 milligram of iron per day. In menstruating women, the reserve is not more than 200–400 milligrams, but iron losses average 1.5 milligrams per day, and sometimes as much as 2.4 milligrams per day. In a study of female college students, only six out of the seventy-four studied (about 12 percent) were getting the RDA for iron. Other surveys have shown that 10–30 percent of the women studied have iron deficits. The RDA for women (18 milligrams) is nearly twice as high as that for men (10 milligrams). Yet women and girls have lower caloric requirements and consequently *cannot* supply their needs even when they follow a diet of carefully selected foods.

Some researchers have expressed concern that vegetarian women may be at an even higher risk than nonvegetarians for low iron intake. Based on an actual analysis of their diet, the average intake was 11–14 milligrams per day for lacto-ovo vegetarian women. This is below the RDA; however, nonvegetarian women appear to have similar low intakes.

Pregnant women are at particularly high risk for low iron, with deficiencies as high as 60 percent. I usually recommend supplements for these women because their needs are not met by the average diet. They often have had a marginal iron intake before becoming pregnant, and therefore their iron stores are below optimum, putting themselves and their babies at risk.

Achlorhydria (low stomach acid), removal of part of the stomach, and malabsorption syndromes have been shown to reduce iron absorption. In addition, calcium phosphate salts, tannic acid in tea, and antacids tend to interfere with iron absorption. Phytates, a substance found in high-fiber foods, may interfere with iron absorption; however, this evidence is inconclusive.

Food Sources: Foods that are highest in iron are meat (especially liver), poultry, and fish. Other substantial sources are eggs, breads and cereals (either whole grain or enriched with iron), leafy vegetables, potatoes and other vegetables, fruit, and milk.

The absorbability of iron from foods varies widely. The "organic" iron found in red meats is the most absorbable (10–30 percent). Plants contain "inorganic" iron, only 2–10 percent of which is absorbed by our digestive tracts. In addition, large quantities of iron are lost from food that is cooked in water that is then discarded. However, when you cook acidic foods in cast-iron cookware, iron from the cookware leaches out into the foods, increasing its iron content considerably. In addition, vitamin C enhances the absorbability of iron in nonanimal foods.

OPTIMUM DAILY ALLOWANCE—ODA

For optimum general health, the basic Optimum Daily Allowance for iron is:

15–25 mg for men
20–30 mg for women

In my clinical experience, I have found the following amounts of iron to be valuable for:

Iron deficiency anemia . . . . 20–30 mg
Chronic fatigue . . . . 15–20 mg
Poor attention span . . . . 15–20 mg

Remember: If you have a medical condition, please consult your physician before taking supplements.

Anemia due to iron deficiency will respond fairly rapidly, but supplements should be continued for several months to fully replenish the body stores. You should be aware that anemia may also be due to a vitamin B-12 or folic acid deficiency. Other possible causes of anemia are internal bleeding, adverse effects of certain drugs, and the presence of toxins in the body. There is a condition called "sports anemia" which is not a true anemia. It is due to abnormal destruction of red blood cells due to mechanical injury, not to inadequate iron, and so routine iron supplementation is not justified. Be sure to consult with your doctor if you show signs of anemia.

SUPPLEMENTS

Iron is available as an individual supplement and as a part of many vitamin-mineral formulas. The most common form is iron sulphate, which is very inexpensive but can be irritating to the digestive tract. I recommend iron fumarate and iron gluconate since they are less irritating to the digestive tract and less likely to cause constipation. As with the other minerals, look for the "elemental" iron content when buying supplements.

TOXICITY AND ADVERSE EFFECTS

The toxicity of iron is low; harmful effects of daily intakes of up to 75 milligrams per day are unlikely in healthy persons. We have a highly effective mechanism that prevents an overload of iron from entering our bodies and causing toxicity. The amount of iron our bodies absorb is carefully regulated by the intestines according to our bodies' needs. The greater our need, the higher the rate of absorption. Growing children, pregnant women, and anemic individuals have higher rates of absorption. When a deficiency occurs, the rate of absorption increases to two to three times more than normal. (Unfortunately, this response does not appear to be sufficient to prevent anemia in iron-deficient subjects who are only mildly anemic and whose iron intake is marginal.)

However, it is possible yet very rare to have too much iron. A disease called hemosiderosis is a disorder of iron metabolism in which large amounts of iron are deposited in the body, especially in the liver, but sometimes also in the lungs, pancreas, and heart. It was originally discovered in the Bantu tribes in South Africa, who ingest as much as 100 milligrams of iron per day, and has also been known to occur following prolonged unnecessary iron therapy. Although there was some early evidence that iron supplements might compromise zinc status, the results of subsequent studies have been contradictory.

Chapter 26

COPPER

The average adult has about 100–150 milligrams of copper in the body. It is stored in the liver, brain, heart, and kidney and is found in the hair. Copper helps your body absorb and use iron to synthesize hemoglobin. It also plays a role in maintaining the integrity of myelin (the outer covering of the nerves). Copper is needed for taste sensitivity, the maturation of collagen, the formation of elastin, and bone development. It is a constituent of a number of enzymes required for energy production, the oxidation of fatty acids, and the formation of melanin, a skin pigment. Copper is also involved in the metabolism of ascorbic acid.

Symptoms of copper deficiency in animals are anemia, skeletal defects, degeneration of the nervous system, defects in the pigmentation and structure of the hair, reproductive problems, and abnormalities in the cardiovascular system. Mild copper deficiency in animals has resulted in an elevated serum cholesterol, especially when the zinc intake is high. Copper supplements have been shown to lower total cholesterol and raise HDL cholesterol (the "good" kind) in experimental animals and humans who have copper deficiency.

Abnormally high blood copper levels are often seen in people with viral infections, rheumatoid arthritis, rheumatic fever, lupus erythematosis, myocardial infarction, leukemia, and certain cancers, although the causes for the increased levels of copper are unexplained. It may be that excess copper plays a role in the development and progression of these diseases, or it may be that the body is circulating more copper in an attempt to deal with the diseases. When experimental animals were given oral contraceptives, their blood copper levels were significantly elevated.

Drugs containing copper complexes have been shown to be effective in combating many inflammatory diseases including rheumatoid arthritis, osteoarthritis, ankylosing spondylitis, rheumatic fever, and sciatica. They are also useful in the treatment of ulcers, convulsions, chorea, cancer, and diabetes. These are diseases of specific tissues that need to be repaired. It is thought that the drugs' positive effects are due to the copper complexes' ability to facilitate or promote tissue repair processes that use copper-dependent enzymes.

Copper plays a role in the immune system. Experimentally induced copper *deficiencies* or *excesses* have each been reported to increase the severity of a wide variety of infections in laboratory animals.

There is no RDA for copper. Copper is so widely available in foods and through the use of copper cooking utensils that deficiency in this mineral is thought to be rare in humans. Many believe that even a diet that is poor in other nutrients is likely to furnish enough copper. However, recent research suggests the typical American diet may not contain the amount of copper it was originally thought to contain (see "Food Sources," below). In addition, there are some groups who are at particular risk of suboptimal copper intake.

Deficiency may occur in severely malnourished individuals, in which case the symptoms are anemia, impaired immunity, and bone disease. Similar symptoms have also been detected in premature infants who were fed an exclusive diet of cow's milk, which is low in copper. People who suffer from sprue or celiac disease may have difficulty absorbing copper. The chronic use of certain antacids can deplete the body of copper, and should be considered as a risk factor. There is evidence that an excess of zinc may interfere with copper absorption, which may increase the requirements for copper. Pregnant women may be at risk. In a study that looked at twenty-four healthy women during their pregnancy, the copper intake from their diet was way below normal, and even when supplements brought the daily total intake up to 2.7 milligrams per day, this was marginal in meeting their needs. Research has demonstrated that a copper deficiency in pregnant animals may cause birth defects in their offspring.

Food Sources: Copper is widely distributed in foods, with liver, shellfish, meats, nuts, legumes, whole grain cereals, and raisins being the richest sources. Early data indicate that the average dietary intake of copper is 2–5 milligrams. However, more recent surveys indicate a much lower intake, often substantially below 1 milligram per day. We don't know whether this discrepancy is due to an actual decline in copper intake or differences in measuring techniques. Another factor to consider is that only 25 percent of the copper ingested is absorbed, and that many people eat highly processed, demineralized foods. Drinking water may contribute to your total daily copper intake, but this varies with the type of piping and hardness of water.

OPTIMUM DAILY ALLOWANCE—ODA

For optimum general health, the Optimum Daily Allowance for copper is:

0.5–2 mg for men and women

There is not enough data for me to make recommendations for specific conditions and concerns at this time. For most individuals the zinc-to-copper ratio can range from 10:1 to 15:1. For example, if you ingest 30 milligrams of zinc per day, and 2 milligrams copper a day, your zinc to copper ratio would be 15:1. I recommend using these ratios to figure how much copper to consume. If you consume larger quantities of copper, or are taking certain drugs or have a disorder that actually requires the lowering of your copper level, you should consult with a professional who may advise against copper supplementation.

WARNING: If you suffer from Wilson's disease, please do not take a copper supplement (see "Toxicity and Adverse Effects," below).

Remember: If you have a medical condition, please consult with your physician before taking supplements.

SUPPLEMENTS

Copper is available as an individual supplement and is often included in multivitamin-mineral formulas. Copper gluconate is the form I recommend since copper sulphate can be irritating to the digestive tract.

TOXICITY AND ADVERSE EFFECTS

Copper toxicity occurs in a hereditary disorder called Wilson's disease. The symptoms are hepatitis, degeneration of the lens of the eye, kidney malfunction, and neurological disorders. Acute excessive doses of copper produces nausea, vomiting, abdominal pains, diarrhea, headache, dizziness, and a metallic taste in the mouth. When untreated, it may lead to death.

Chapter 27

MANGANESE

Most of the information about manganese comes from animal experiments. When this is combined with some human data, it appears that this mineral has many important uses in the body. Manganese is an essential part of many enzyme systems involved in protein, fat, and energy metabolism. It is needed for normal bone growth and development and for normal reproduction. Studies have implicated low manganese levels in human infants with birth defects ranging from cleft palate to bone deformities.

Manganese is required for the proper functioning of the nerves. Animals fed manganese-deficient diets show an increased susceptibility to convulsions. There is also some evidence that insufficient manganese may exacerbate a tendency to have epileptic seizures, according to a study involving young human patients.

Experiments have yielded evidence suggesting that manganese deficiencies may affect the immune system. Antibody response and the activity of microphages, granulocytes, and phagocytes are all stimulated by manganese. In addition, manganese is a component of the enzyme superoxide dismutase (SOD). SOD prevents the free radical damage that is implicated in the degeneration of tissues associated with the aging process, and with cell changes that may lead to cancer.

Experiments indicate that manganese deficiency may play a role in glucose tolerance. In one animal study, for example, the insulin output in response to glucose of rats who were deficient in this mineral was 76 to 63 percent of the insulin output of manganese-sufficient rats. It has also been reported that oral manganese supplements significantly lowered blood glucose levels in a patient who was unresponsive to insulin. These data have exciting implications for people with blood sugar problems.

There is no established RDA for manganese. There is only the Food and Nutrition Board's recommendation that we consume approximately 2.5–5 milligrams daily. This amount is roughly what one would consume if one were eating the typical American highly refined diet. However, some researchers have noted that diets high in milk and refined carbohydrates may not supply adequate manganese. There is an especially high risk of deficiency when manganese requirements are increased, as during pregnancy or times of rapid growth.

In view of the fact that manganese is poorly absorbed and is severely lacking in refined foods, I and many practitioners feel that the recommendation for manganese is much too low. The recommendation of 2.5–5 milligrams per day is based on what people *are* consuming, not what they *should* be consuming.

Food Sources: Good sources of manganese include nuts and seeds (especially hazelnuts and pecans), avocado, seaweed, and whole grains such as oatmeal, buckwheat, and whole wheat. Other fruits and vegetables contain moderate amounts. Refined grains are a poor source of manganese: Milling removes 73 percent of this trace element, and the enrichment process does not put it back.

In general, the manganese in food is poorly absorbed in the intestine. It appears that phytates (substances found in plant fiber) in particular interfere with manganese absorption. However, it is probable that this effect occurs to a significant degree only when extremely high amounts of fiber are eaten.

OPTIMUM DAILY ALLOWANCE—ODA

For optimum general health, the basic Optimum Daily Allowance for manganese is:

15–30 mg for men and women

In my clinical experience, I have found the following amounts of manganese to be valuable for:

Impaired glucose tolerance . . . . 20–30 mg
Cancer prevention . . . . 15–30 mg

Remember: If you have a medical condition, please consult with your physician before taking supplements.

SUPPLEMENTS

Manganese is available in individual supplements and in some multivita-min-mineral formulas. Manganese gluconate and chelated manganese are the forms I recommend.

TOXICITY AND ADVERSE EFFECTS

The toxicity for manganese is low when it is ingested either in the form of manganese-rich foods or manganese supplements. Toxicity does exist when manganese is inhaled. This occurs in the cases of certain miners who are exposed to high concentrations of manganese oxide in the air on the job. In these cases, even small doses can cause psychiatric abnormalities and nerve disorders.

Chapter 28

CHROMIUM

As adults, our bodies contain approximately 6 grams of chromium. It is most highly concentrated in the hair, spleen, kidney and testes. The heart, pancreas, lungs, and brain also contain this trace mineral, but in lower concentrations.

Chromium activates many enzymes involved in the metabolism of glucose and the synthesis of proteins. Glucose, commonly known as blood sugar, is the fuel the cells of our body "burns" for energy. Insulin is the hormone that regulates the amount of glucose in our blood. It "escorts" glucose into our cells so it can be stored for later use, preventing our blood sugar from going too high (diabetes) or too low (hypoglycemia). Chromium is the major mineral involved in insulin production. It therefore should come as no surprise that a lack of this mineral interferes with insulin production and utilization. There is strong and growing evidence that many disorders in glucose metabolism, namely diabetes and hypoglycemia, may actually be chromium deficiency states. In experiments, chromium supplementation has actually been found to improve glucose tolerance in some diabetics and people with impaired glucose tolerance.

In one study for example, ten elderly individuals were given chromium supplementation. In four of them, all abnormal features of the glucose tolerance test (GTT) disappeared. These "chromium responders" had had mild abnormalities of the GTT, but the "nonresponders" had more severe abnormalities. This, combined with the pattern of response, suggests that the nonresponders might have been so severely deficient in chromium that it would have taken longer for them to show any improvement. When I have given GTF chromium to adult-onset diabetics, along with a diet and exercise program, their physicians were able to reduce their insulin injections or oral medications. In addition, many patients on this regimen are able to stop insulin and oral medications completely.

Chromium depletion has also been implicated in hypercholesterolemia (high cholesterol in the blood), again because of its role in insulin production and glucose regulation. Glucose is the primary source of energy for the body, so if chromium depletion results in ineffective insulin and seriously impaired glucose metabolism, then the body must rely on lipid (fat) metabolism for energy. This is a less-than-satisfactory situation because some of the by-products of lipid metabolism are made into cholesterol. Many researchers believe that the accelerated atherosclerosis seen in diabetics may be due to this process. In fact, studies have shown that chromium deficiency tends to decrease the liver's uptake of cholesterol and fatty acids, which could favor the accumulation of lipids in the arteries. In laboratory experiments, rats fed a chromium-deficient high-sugar diet showed a dramatically increased accumulation of cholesterol in the arteries. On the other hand, when rats fed a high-sugar diet were supplemented with chromium, it significantly lowered their serum cholesterol levels and resulted in less accumulation of lipids in the arteries. There is epidemiological evidence too: In several Oriental nations where low serum cholesterol levels are frequently found, these same populations have relatively high chromium concentrations in tissue. Other studies have shown that chromium supplements increase HDL cholesterol (the "good" cholesterol) in addition to lowering overall cholesterol.

There is no established RDA for chromium. According to long-term studies in human subjects, 200–290 micrograms are required daily in order to maintain a balance or near-balance of chromium. However, the estimated chromium intake for the average American is 50–100 micrograms per day. This is lower than in Italy, Egypt, South America, and India. Even a diet that is considered to be adequate in other respects may be marginal in chromium, and chromium deficiency is believed to be relatively common in the United States and other developed countries. This is no doubt due at least in part to the refining of grains, which removes over three quarters of the chromium. (We already learned in Chapter 27 that refining removes 73 percent of the manganese. It is interesting to note that a lack of both of these minerals has been implicated in diabetes.)

Athletes may be at risk for marginal chromium deficiency. Strenuous running places considerable stress on the body and increases the energy requirements by seven to twenty times. This results in changes in hormones and other substances that function in glucose metabolism.

Food Sources: Brewer's yeast, beer, meat (especially liver), cheese, and whole grain cereals and breads are good sources of chromium. Leafy vegetables contain chromium, but it is poorly absorbed. White rice and white bread are poor sources of this mineral. The milling of grains removes up to 83 percent of the chromium, and none of this is replaced during the enrichment process.

OPTIMUM DAILY ALLOWANCE—ODA

For optimum general health, the basic Optimum Daily Allowance for chromium is:

200–600 mcg for men and women

In my clinical experience, I have found the following amounts of GTF chromium to be valuable for:

Impaired glucose tolerance . . . . 400–600 mcg
High cholesterol . . . . 200–400 mcg

Remember: If you have a medical condition, please consult with your physician before taking supplements.

SUPPLEMENTS

Chromium is available as an individual supplement and as a component of some multivitamin-mineral formulas. GTF (Glucose Tolerance Factor) chromium is the form I recommend since it is the most absorbable form. It is chromium combined with glycine, glutamic acid, cysteine, and niacin.

TOXICITY AND ADVERSE EFFECTS

There is no known toxicity for chromium, except in the case of chromium miners and industrial exposure where chromium dust is inhaled.

Chapter 29

SELENIUM

Selenium is present in all the tissues of the body, but is concentrated most highly in the kidney, liver, spleen, pancreas, and testes.

People do not take in enough selenium both because of the type of diet they eat and because of the low selenium content of the soil in which their food was grown or raised. The soil content of selenium varies widely, with many areas showing serious depletion. In fact, there have been several reports of selenium deficiencies in livestock that were raised where the selenium content of the soil is low. Their symptoms include abnormalities in the vascular system, cataracts, hair loss, and degeneration of the pancreas.

In humans, there is evidence that inadequate selenium is involved in heart disease. Overt deficiencies have been found in alcoholics with cirrhosis of the liver, and in people who have been receiving long-term intravenous feeding. These people suffered from heart problems which responded to selenium supplementation. In eastern Finland, which has one of the highest mortality rates from heart disease in the world, it was found that low selenium in the blood was associated with up to a six to sevenfold increase in the risk of death from heart disease. In addition, children in certain areas of China where the selenium content of the soil is low develop a heart disease called Keshan's disease. Their heart problems respond to selenium supplements.

There is some evidence that selenium may also prove effective in the treatment or prevention of several other problems. A study using 400 micrograms of selenium and approximately 25 IU of vitamin E markedly improved skin conditions such as acne and seborrheic dermatitis. A Danish study examined patients with rheumatoid arthritis and found that they had lower levels of selenium. Those with the lowest levels had the more severe form of this disease. Another fascinating study conducted in Scandinavia showed a correlation between low selenium levels and the incidence and severity of muscular dystrophy; one patient who was treated with selenium supplements showed considerable improvement after one year. Finnish researchers have also conducted a study on elderly patients who were given large doses of selenium and vitamin E for one year. They found an obvious improvement after two months in their patients' mental well-being including less fatigue, depression, and anxiety and more mental alertness, motivation, and self-care. A recent study conducted in Japan suggests that selenium and vitamin E may enhance the responsiveness of arthritis patients to conventional treatment.

Recent studies have shown that people with celiac disease are at high risk for low selenium, either because their low gluten diets are low in selenium, or because of problems with absorption. Down's Syndrome patients have also been found to have low levels of selenium. Exposure to certain environmental chemicals may increase the requirements for selenium. For example, oil refinery workers were found to have low selenium levels, in spite of their dietary intake of 217 micrograms per day, which is over the safe and adequate range of 50–200 micrograms established by the Food and Nutrition Board. Selenium has been shown to be effective in protecting against the toxic effects of mercury poisoning, which can occur with environmental exposure to mercury, such as in dentistry.

However, selenium's best-known and perhaps most important biological function relates to its role as an antioxidant and anticancer mineral. As we have seen in other chapters, free radicals damage our cells and may lead to the development of cancer. Selenium is a component of the enzyme glutathione peroxidase, which protects our cells against this damage. Many animal studies have proved that selenium deficiencies increase the incidence and rate of growth of cancers in animals when they were either exposed to a variety of potent carcinogens or received transplanted tumors. Companion studies have shown that high selenium intake protects against these cancers. For example, in one study in which rats were exposed to a potent carcinogen, only 15 percent of those who were also given selenium developed liver cancer, as compared with 90 percent of unsupplemented rats. In another study, the occurrence of cancer was 10 percent versus 80 percent. In yet another animal study, selenium supplementation reduced the colon cancer incidence by more than 50 percent.

In humans, there is ample epidemiological evidence that high selenium is correlated with a lower incidence of many types of cancer. Researchers have found that cancer risk is reduced in people living in areas with selenium-rich soil, in people with a high-selenium food supply, and in people with higher blood levels of selenium. Selenium intakes in the groups of people studied were close to 750 micrograms per day with no toxic side effects noted. In a survey that spanned twenty-seven countries including the United States, it was found that the cancer death rate was lower in those people whose typical diets were high in selenium. The cancers involved in this and similar studies indicate that selenium appears to be especially protective against cancer of the breast, colon, and lung. Data also suggest protection against tumors of the ovary, cervix, rectum, bladder, esophagus, pancreas, skin, liver, and prostate, as well as leukemia.

It has been known since 1969 that the blood levels of cancer patients are low in selenium. In general, cancer patients with lower-than-average selenium levels have more multiple primary tumors, multiple recurrences, distant metastases, and a shortened survival time. In a study of twelve thousand people conducted in Finland, the risk of fatal cancer was nearly six times as high in people with the lowest serum selenium compared to those with the highest concentrations.

In several studies, it has been shown that selenium and vitamin E (and perhaps vitamin A) have a synergistic effect. An example of this may be found in the Finnish study mentioned earlier. In this study, male smokers who died of cancer had lower serum selenium, vitamin A, and vitamin E levels than the healthy controls. It is well known that vitamin E enhances the antioxidant effect of selenium. Supplementation with selenium alone and with selenium plus vitamin E in excess of the established quantities has been found to stimulate the immune system in experimental animals. This effect was particularly pronounced when the diet was high in polyunsaturated fats (PUFA). A diet high in PUFA has been linked to a higher incidence of certain cancers.

These studies show promise for the prevention and possible treatment of cancer with selenium supplementation. When combined with other supplements, the anticancer effect may be even more pronounced. "Chemopreventive" trials of several nutrients including selenium, vitamin E, and vitamin A are now being conducted by the National Cancer Institute. However, these trials are unfortunately limited to 200 micrograms per day, which may be too low a dose to observe the full potential protective effect of this mineral. Larger doses of selenium have been shown to be protective in animals, and safe in humans. In addition, we are not sure to what extent selenium supplementation influences the later stages of carcinogenesis. If its influence is strongest in the early stage, it will be very difficult for these trials to prove the connection between low selenium and cancer because of the long latency period for most cancers. (For example, it may take up to fourteen years for a single breast cancer cell to multiply and produce a tumor large enough to be detected by currently available diagnostic methods.) Finally, evidence of the synergism of nutrients has led many researchers to emphasize the need to consider several nutrients in diet and cancer studies instead of focusing on just one nutrient per study.

Food Sources: There are no accurate measurements of the selenium content of foods available. However, it appears that the richest sources of selenium are seafoods, organ meats, and meat, if the animals of origin ate a diet high in selenium. Whole grains can be good sources, but similarly this depends upon the selenium content of the soil in which they are grown. Fruits and vegetables generally contain very low amounts of selenium.

The refining process strips foods of their selenium content. In one study, it was found that a highly refined diet contains 61 percent less selenium than a diet rich in unrefined foods. Cooking also reduces the content significantly, especially if the cooking water is discarded. Vitamin C seems to enhance the absorption of selenium.

OPTIMUM DAILY ALLOWANCE—ODA

For optimum general health, the basic Optimum Daily Allowance for selenium is:

100–400 mcg for men and women living in low-selenium areas (These include coastal areas and glaciated areas.)

50–200 mcg for men and women living in high-selenium areas

In my clinical experience, I have found the following amounts of selenium to be valuable for:

Cancer prevention . . . . 200–400 mcg

Heart disease . . . . 100–300 mcg

Mercury accumulation . . . . 50–200 mcg

Arthritis . . . . 50–400 mcg

Remember: If you have a medical condition, please consult with your physician before taking supplements.

SUPPLEMENTS

Selenium is most often available as an individual supplement, although some multivitamin-mineral formulas are beginning to include it, generally in small amounts. I recommend selenium in the form of selenomethionine, extracted from selenium-rich yeast or ocean plants. This form is the least toxic and appears to be the most absorbable.

TOXICITY AND ADVERSE EFFECTS

Animal poisoning due to high-selenium soil is well known. The evidence so far seems to indicate that for toxicity to occur in humans the intake must be very high indeed. Various studies have shown that long-term intakes of up to 500–750 micrograms per day have produced no signs of toxicity in humans. Data extrapolated from animal studies suggest that toxicity does not occur in humans ingesting less than 1000–2000 micrograms per day. The Food and Nutrition Board has stated that overt selenium toxicity may occur in humans ingesting 2400–3000 micrograms daily. (But for some reason the Board still claims the maximum intake of selenium should not exceed 200 micrograms.) Toxicity symptoms include a garlic odor in breath, urine, and sweat and have been reported among people living in high-selenium areas and among certain workers exposed to selenium. Some data, when combined with selenium's known teratogenic effect in animals, suggest that extremely high levels of selenium may also cause birth defects in humans.

Chapter 30

IODINE

We contain about 20–30 milligrams of iodine in our bodies. Approximately three quarters of this is found in our thyroid, and the remainder is distributed throughout the body, mostly in the fluid that bathes our cells.

Iodine, therefore, is important for the proper functioning of the thyroid gland. It is a necessary constituent of the thyroid hormones used to regulate our metabolism. These hormones influence physical and mental growth, the functioning of the nervous system and muscles, circulatory activity, and the metabolism of all nutrients.

The classic iodine deficiency disease is goiter. This is a condition during which the thyroid gland becomes enormously enlarged in an effort to compensate for insufficient hormone production. If the thyroid cannot overcome this insufficiency, symptoms of listlessness, lassitude, and sluggishness appear. Goiter may also appear in people who ingest large amounts of goitrogens, substances which decrease the production of a thyroid hormone. Goitrogenic foods include rutabagas, strawberries, peaches, cabbage, peanuts, spinach, and radishes.

The Recommended Daily Allowance for iodine is 150 micrograms for adults; 175 micrograms and 200 micrograms for pregnant and lactating women, respectively. The estimated intake in the United States is between 64 and 677 micrograms per day. Areas in the United States where iodine deficiency is most common are called "goiter belts" and include the Midwest, the Pacific Northwest, and the Great Lakes region. Switzerland, Central America, the mountainous regions of South America, New Zealand, and the Himalayas also suffer a high incidence of goiter owing to low-iodine soil. Simple goiter is found most often in women, especially during adolescence, pregnancy, and menopause.

Since the introduction of iodized table salt, the incidence of goiter has fallen dramatically. A survey revealed that the rates in Michigan and Texas were approximately 5 to 6 percent. It remains to be seen whether the recent efforts to cut down on salt consumption will have any effect on the goiter incidence.

Recent data indicate that there may be other uses for iodine. For example, the results of a study of iodine-deficient children in China suggest that hearing loss may be an iodine deficiency disorder. In addition, there is growing interest in using iodine supplements in the event of a nuclear accident to prevent the absorption of radioactive iodine by the thyroid to protect against thyroid damage, and possibly thyroid cancer.

Food Sources: The richest and most consistent food sources of iodine are seafoods, including fish, shellfish, and plants. Seaweed is incredibly high in iodine, and can have as much as 50,000 micrograms per 3 ounces. Most land vegetables are rather low in iodine, unless they are grown near the seacoast, or have been fertilized with iodine-containing fertilizers. The iodine content of meat, dairy products, and eggs depends upon the iodine content of the animals' diet. Livestock destined for consumption may be encouraged to lick salt blocks that contain iodine so their meat will be higher in this mineral. For many individuals, the most important dietary source of iodine is iodized salt, 1 gram of which supplies about 76 micrograms of iodine.

OPTIMUM DAILY ALLOWANCE—ODA

For optimum general health, the basic Optimum Daily Allowance for iodine is:

150–300 mcg for men and women

50–150 mcg for men and women who routinely consume iodized salt and/or seaweed

Remember: If you have a medical condition, please consult your physician. If you are allergic to iodine you may need to avoid this mineral.

SUPPLEMENTS

Many individuals are supplemented with iodine through the use of iodized table salt. However, if you do not wish to increase your consumption of salt, iodine is also available in tablets as "sea kelp" and in concentrated liquid drops. The iodine available for medicinal use is not to be used orally because it is poisonous.

TOXICITY AND ADVERSE EFFECTS

An intake of up to 1000 micrograms of iodine per day is considered safe. Toxicity symptoms include rash, headache, difficulty in breathing, and a metallic taste in the mouth. Very high doses (20,000 micrograms per day) can paradoxically cause a form of goiter called "iodide goiter." This has been seen in certain groups of Japanese who consume great quantities of seaweed daily.

Chapter 31

POTASSIUM

Our cells contain more potassium than any other mineral; as adults, we are comprised of a total of approximately 250 grams. Potassium is essential in maintaining the fluid balance in our cells and is required for the enzymatic reactions taking place within them. Potassium is used to convert glucose into glycogen for storage. It is used for nerve transmission, contraction of muscles, hormone secretion, and other functions.

Potassium deficiency symptoms include nausea, vomiting (which can ironically lead to further potassium losses), listlessness, feelings of apprehension, muscle weakness, muscle spasms and cramps, tachycardia (rapid heartbeat), and in extreme cases, heart failure.

There is a growing body of evidence that low levels of potassium are associated with high blood pressure and deserve more attention. This association may be especially strong when the sodium-to-potassium ratio is high. Some researchers feel, in fact, that low potassium may play a more significant role in hypertension than high sodium does in some individuals. In one study, for example, some hypertensives responded to sodium restriction and others to potassium supplementation. As some researchers point out, diets restricted in calories, sodium, and cholesterol are often recommended to people with cardiovascular disease. It is ironic that such diets also increase the risk of reducing nutrients such as calcium and potassium that may be essential for maintaining normal blood pressure.

Potassium may prove to be of value to the cardiovascular system in other ways. In an animal study, rats were given stroke-inducing diets. The group that was supplemented with potassium suffered a 2 percent rate of fatal strokes, as compared with 83 percent in the unsupplemented group. In another animal study, potassium supplementation was able to protect against the kidney damage resulting from hypertension. In both these studies, these remarkable effects occurred even when potassium did not reduce blood pressure.

There is no Recommended Daily Allowance for potassium. It has been estimated that the average American diet contains from 2 to 6 grams per day. Potassium deficiency can result from severe malnutrition, alcoholism, anorexia nervosa, vomiting, or diarrhea, and in illnesses that seriously interfere with the appetite. Potassium may be depleted following severe tissue injury due to surgery and burns, and during prolonged fevers. The excessive use of steroids, laxatives, and some diuretics also encourage potassium losses from the body. If a person already has heart disease, low potassium can worsen the picture. Hypertensives who are taking diuretics under a doctor's care are often given potassium supplements to counteract this effect.

Potassium must exist in a balance with sodium in the body. Although sodium may be an important dietary determinant of blood pressure, variations in the potassium-to-sodium ratio in the diet affect the blood pressure under certain circumstances. So when considering potassium levels, we must consider sodium levels as well and watch out for hidden high-sodium foods, including processed foods such as canned goods, luncheon meats, sausages, and frozen foods.

Food Sources: Potassium is widely distributed in foods. Dairy products (except for cheese, because potassium is lost in the whey), meats, poultry, and fish are good sources; legumes, fruits, vegetables, and whole grains are also respectable sources. People with high blood pressure on diuretics are frequently advised to eat fruits such as bananas, oranges, and tomatoes for their potassium content. However, recent evidence indicates that the retention of potassium in these foods is poor. In addition, even if all the potassium in bananas were retained, it would take an enormous number of bananas per day to provide the recommended amount of potassium for a patient taking diuretics.

Bear in mind, too, that potassium is lost through cooking. A boiled potato may have lost up to 50 percent of its original potassium content; a steamed potato, only 3 to 6 percent. Some researchers have suggested adding modest amounts of salt substitute containing potassium chloride to boiling water to prevent the potassium from leaching out during cooking.

OPTIMUM DAILY ALLOWANCE—ODA

Since potassium is so easily available in fresh foods, most people do not require a potassium supplement. Rather, most people should be advised to reduce sodium intake so a more favorable sodium-to-potassium ratio is achieved. If, however, you wish to take a supplement, the Optimum Daily Allowance of potassium is:

99–300 mg for men and women

Higher levels of potassium may be suggested by your physician if you are taking certain diuretics.

Remember: If you have a medical condition, please consult with your physician before taking supplements.

SUPPLEMENTS

Potassium is available in tablet and liquid form. Levels above the ODA should be taken only under the advice of a professional.

TOXICITY AND ADVERSE EFFECTS

Potassium toxicity is seen when daily intakes exceed 18 grams, an amount that is unlikely to be ingested through food. Toxicity usually occurs only through the uneducated use of supplements, or when an individual has kidney failure. Excess potassium may cause muscle fatigue, irregular heartbeat, and possibly heart failure.

PART FOUR

APPENDIXES AND NOTES

QUICK-REFERENCE CHART
FOR THE VITAMINS AND MINERALS

*THE BASIC OPTIMUM DAILY ALLOWANCE (ODA) is for general health and disease prevention. Some individuals may wish to use higher levels, depending upon risk factors such as pollution, stress, personal and family health history.

NUTRIENT	MAJOR USES	FOOD SOURCES	RDA	BASIC ODA
Vitamin A; beta-carotene	Prevents night blindness; other eye problems May be useful for acne; other skin disorders Enhances immunity Cancer prevention May heal gastrointestinal ulcers Protects against pollution Needed for epithelial tissue maintenance and repair	Fish liver oils, animal livers, green and yellow fruits and vegetables	4000–5000 IU	10,000–75,000 IU (in a mixture of A and beta carotene)
Vitamin D	Required for calcium and phosphorus absorption and utilization Prevention and treatment of osteoporosis Enhances immunity	Fish liver oils, fatty saltwater fish, Vitamin D-fortified dairy products, eggs	400 IU	400–600 IU
Vitamin E	Antioxidant Cancer prevention Cardiovascular disease prevention Improves circulation Tissue repair May prevent age spots Useful in treating fibrocystic breasts Useful in treating PMS	Cold-pressed vegetable oils, whole grains, dark-green leafy vegetables, nuts, legumes	10–20 IU	200–800 IU
Vitamin K	Needed for blood clotting May play a role in bone formation May prevent osteoporosis	Green leafy vegetables	None established	

NUTRIENT	MAJOR USES	FOOD SOURCES	RDA	BASIC ODA*
B Complex				
B-1 (thiamin); B-2 (ribo-flavin); B-3 (niacin/amide); B-6 (pyri-doxine)	Maintain healthy nerves, skin, eyes, hair, liver, mouth, muscle tone in gastrointestinal tract B vitamins are coenzymes involved in energy production Emotional or physical stress increases need May be useful for depression or anxiety	Unrefined whole grains, liver, green leafy vegetables, fish, poultry, eggs, meat, nuts, beans	Ranges from 1.2–14 mg	25–300 mg

B-1: High-carbohydrate diet increases need.
B-2: May be useful with B-6 for treatment of carpal tunnel syndrome. May prevent cataracts. Increased need with oral contraceptives. Increased need with strenuous exercise.
B-3: Useful for circulatory problems. Lowers serum cholesterol and triglycerides.
B-6: May be useful in preventing oxalate stones. May be used as mild diuretic. May be useful for PMS. Increased need with oral contraceptives. May be useful in treating asthma.

B-12 (cobalamin)	Needed for fat and carbohydrate metabolism Prevention and treatment of B-12 anemia Maintains proper nervous system function May be useful for anxiety and depression	Kidney, liver, egg, herring, mackerel, milk, cheese, tofu, seafood	3 mcg	25–300 mcg
Folic acid	Works closely with B-12 Involved in protein metabolism Needed for healthy cell division and replication Prevention and treatment of folic acid anemia Stress may increase need May be useful for depression and anxiety May be useful in treating cervical dysplasia Oral contraceptives may increase need	Beef, lamb, pork, chicken liver, green leafy vegetables, whole wheat, bran, yeast	400 mcg	400–1200 mcg

(continued on next page)

NUTRIENT	MAJOR USES	FOOD SOURCES	RDA	BASIC ODA*
Pantothenic acid	Needed in fat, protein, and carbohydrate metabolism Needed for synthesis of hormones and cholesterol Needed for red blood cell production Needed for nerve transmission Vital for healthy function of the adrenal glands May be useful for joint inflammation May be useful for depression and anxiety	Eggs, salt water fish, pork, beef, milk, whole wheat, beans, fresh vegetables	None	25–300 mg
Biotin	Needed for metabolism of protein, fats, and carbohydrates Not enough data available, but deficiencies may be implicated in high serum cholesterol, seborrheic dermatitis, and certain nervous system disorders	Meat, cooked egg yolk, poultry, yeast, soy beans, milk, salt water fish, whole grains	None	25–300 mcg
Choline and Inositol	Involved in metabolism of fat and cholesterol, fat absorption and utilization Choline makes an important brain neurotransmitter	Egg yolk, whole grains, vegetables, organ meats, fruits, milk	None	25–300 mg
PABA	Needed for protein metabolism Needed for folic acid metabolism Used topically as a sunscreen	Liver, kidney, whole grains, molasses	None	25–300 mg

Note: A combination of all B vitamins can usually be found in B-complex and multivitamin formulas. If you wish to take any additional B vitamins, please make sure you are taking a complete B complex first.

NUTRIENT	MAJOR USES	FOOD SOURCES	RDA	BASIC ODA*
Vitamin C (ascorbic acid)	Growth and repair of tissues May reduce cholesterol Antioxidant Cancer prevention Enhances immunity Stress increases requirement May reduce high blood pressure May prevent atherosclerosis Protects against pollution	Green vegetables, berries, citrus fruit	60 mg	500–5000 mg (higher during stress or illness)
Calcium	Needed for healthy bones and teeth Needed for nerve transmission Used for muscle function May lower blood pressure Osteoporosis prevention	Dairy foods, salmon, sardines, green leafy vegetables, seafood	800 mg	1000–1500 mg
Phosphorus	Necessary for healthy bones Needed for production of energy Used as a buffering agent Needed for utilization of protein, fats, and carbohydrates	Available in most foods; sodas can be very high	800 mg	Generally available through foods: 200–400 mg
Magnesium	Needed for healthy bones Involved in nerve transmission Needed for muscle function Used in energy formation Needed for healthy blood vessels May lower blood pressure	Widely distributed in foods, especially dairy foods, meat, fish, seafood	300–500 mg	500–750 mg
Zinc	Needed for wound healing Maintains taste and smell acuity Needed for healthy immune system Protects liver from chemical damage	Oysters, fish, seafood, meats, poultry, whole grains, legumes	15 mg	22.5–50 mg

(continued on next page)

NUTRIENT	MAJOR USES	FOOD SOURCES	RDA	BASIC ODA*
Iron	Vital for blood formation Needed for energy production Required for healthy immune system	Meat, poultry, fish, liver, eggs, green leafy vegetables, whole grain or enriched breads and cereals	10-18 mg	15-30 mg
Copper	Involved in blood formation Needed for healthy nerves Needed for taste sensitivity Used in energy production Needed for healthy bone development	Widely distributed in foods, copper cookware, and copper plumbing	None	Needs can generally be met through food: 0.5-2 mg
Manganese	Needed for protein and fat metabolism Used in energy formation Required for normal bone growth and reproduction Needed for healthy nerves Needed for healthy blood sugar regulation Needed for healthy immune system	Nuts, seeds, whole grains, avocado, seaweed	None	15-30 mg
Chromium	Required for glucose metabolism May prevent diabetes May reduce cholesterol	Brewer's yeast, beer, meat, cheese, whole grains	None	200-600 mcg
Selenium	Cancer prevention Heart disease prevention	Depends on soil content, may be in grains and meat	None	50-400 mcg (50-100 mcg for those who live in high-selenium areas)
Iodine	Needed for healthy thyroid gland Prevents goiter	Iodized salts, seafood, saltwater fish, kelp	150 mcg	50-300 mcg (50-150 mcg for those who use iodized salt)
Potassium	May lower blood pressure Needed for energy storage Needed for nerve transmission, muscle contraction, and hormone secretion	Dairy foods, meat, poultry, fish, fruit, legumes, whole grains, vegetables	None	99-300 mg

WORKSHEET

HOW TO USE THE WORKSHEET

Begin by determining your basic ODAs. You may use the basic ODAs given in the worksheet, which are in the low to middle range. They will provide many people with optimum general physical and mental health and will prevent most illnesses. Your own ODAs may differ. The basic ODAs in the individual chapters on vitamins and minerals are given as a dosage range. Based on the information in the individual nutrient chapters and in Part One, decide whether your own ODA should be a low, middle, or high level within this range. Your basic ODAs may be all you need.

However, some people may want to take higher amounts of certain specific nutrients. There may be factors in their lives, such as personal or family health history, which place them at a higher risk for certain diseases and disorders. If you fall into this category, you may want to use supplements to provide an additional margin of safety. The worksheet on pages 170–71 illustrates and summarizes the most frequently encountered of these concerns.

For example, if cancer runs in your family, you would take a higher ODA of the vitamins A, B, C, E; and of the minerals zinc and selenium. If you are concerned about heart disease, your ODAs for vitamin C, vitamin E, and chromium would be higher than the basic ODA. If you have more than one concern, do not add one specific ODA to another; simply use the upper range. For example, if you are concerned about cardiovascular disease prevention and are under great emotional stress, your ODA for vitamin C would be 5000 milligrams, *not* 6000–10,000 milligrams.

If a particular concern of yours is not listed in the worksheet, refer to the individual vitamin and mineral chapters for the ODA range and enter it in one of the columns marked "Other." For example, some women might be concerned about PMS (premenstrual syndrome).

Enter your starting ODA in the worksheet, and date it. As time goes by, evaluate the way you feel and adjust your ODAs accordingly. Always enter and date the adjusted amount in the worksheet so you can keep a working record of your vitamin and mineral program.

SAMPLE WORKSHEET

NUTRIENT	BASIC ODA	EMOTIONAL STRESS	ENHANCE IMMUNITY	CARDIOVASCULAR DISEASE PREVENTION
vit. A	10,000 IU		25,000 – 50,000 IU	
B complex	25 mg	50– 300 mg	50 mg	
vit. C	1000 mg	3000- 5000 mg	5000- 10,000 mg	3000- 5000 mg
vit. D	400 IU			
vit. E	400 IU			400– 800 IU
calcium	1000 mg			
phosphorus	(from diet)			
magnesium	500 mg			
zinc	22.5 mg		50 mg	
copper	2 mg			
manganese	15 mg			
chromium	200 mcg			400 mcg
selenium	100 mcg			
iodine	50– 150 mcg			
potassium	(from diet) (reduce salt)			

CANCER PREVENTION	SKIN PROBLEMS	DIABETES PREVENTION	OSTEOPOROSIS PREVENTION	OTHER	OTHER	YOUR ODA & DATE	YOUR ODA & DATE
50,000 – 100,000 IU	50,000 – 100,000 IU						
50– 150 mg							
5000– 10,000 mg	3000– 5000 mg	1000– 3000 mg					
400 IU			600 IU				
400– 800 IU							
			1500– 2000 mg				
			200– 400 mg				
			750– 2000 mg				
50 mg	50 mg		50 mg				
		30 mg	30 mg				
200 mcg		600 mcg					
400 mcg	200 mcg						

DAILY SUPPLEMENT SCHEDULE AND SHOPPING GUIDE

Use this handy guide when you buy supplements and to help you keep track of your supplement schedule. Make sure to read the labels on your supplements to avoid duplication and double-dosing. For example, if you use a multivitamin supplement with 50 milligrams of B complex, you don't need to take a separate B complex 50. You may, however, want to buy a separate supplement of an individual B vitamin to use for a specific purpose. The same holds true for minerals.

Remember, if you are taking large doses of supplements, they should be divided as evenly as possible throughout the day. Simply write down the number of tablets of each supplement that you take after meals in the appropriate column, and keep the guide displayed for easy reference wherever you store your supplements. (You may want to make a copy of the guide rather than tear it out of the book.) Eventually, taking your supplements will become such a habit you won't need to refer to the schedule. For example, I take my multivitamin-mineral supplement after breakfast and lunch, and take whatever extra individual supplements I need after dinner.

Supplement & Potency	Morning	Afternoon	Evening
vitamin A			
beta-carotene			
B complex			
additional B vitamins:			
vitamin C			
bioflavonoids			
vitamin D			
vitamin E			
calcium			
magnesium			
zinc			
copper			
manganese			
chromium			
selenium			
iodine			
multivitamins			
multiminerals			
other			

REFERENCES

I have drawn on several reference works for much of the background information and overviews on the concepts and nutrients covered in this book. Although they are geared primarily toward the professional, the average reader may also find them of interest:

Bland, Jeffrey. *The Justification for Vitamin Supplementation.* Bellevue, Wash.: Northwest Diagnostic Services, 1981.

Goodhart, Robert S., and Maurice E. Shils. *Modern Nutrition in Health and Disease,* 6th ed. Philadelphia: Lea and Febiger, 1980.

Marks, John. *A Guide to the Vitamins: Their Role in Health and Disease.* Lancaster, Eng.: Medical and Technical Publishing Co., n.d.

The National Research Council. *Recommended Daily Allowances,* 9th ed. Washington, D.C.: National Academy of Sciences, 1980.

Robinson, Corinne H. *Normal and Therapeutic Nutrition,* 15th ed. New York: Macmillan, 1977.

REFERENCE ABSTRACTS FOR THE VITAMIN AND MINERAL CHAPTERS

CHAPTER 6: VITAMIN A

Overviews

Vitamin A is required for vision, reproduction, and maintenance of epithelial tissue. It is beneficial in the treatment of acne, psoriasis, and other skin disorders, and may be important in cancer prevention and in treating precancerous conditions. *The New England Journal of Medicine* 310 (April 19, 1984): 1023–1031.

The authors review evidence regarding the possible mechanisms for the three major recognized functions that are dependent on vitamin A: (1) cell growth and differentiation, (2) reproduction, and (3) vision. *Proceedings of the Society for Experimental Biology and Medicine* 172 (1983): 139–152.

In this study, the vitamin A (and zinc) levels of fifty-four people with Crohn's disease were significantly lower than in nineteen healthy controls. The lower levels did not appear to be caused by malabsorption. The authors conclude that supplementation of these nutrients may be beneficial in patients with highly active Crohn's disease. *Hepatogastroenterology* 32 (January–February 1985): 34–38.

Ulcers

In a four-week study of forty patients with chronic gastric ulcers, the number of patients whose ulcers completely healed or shrank was highest in the group who received 150,000 IU of vitamin A daily. The authors suggest that since gastric ulcer may be thought of as a precancerous condition, vitamin A may have a role in the prevention of cancer from gastric ulcer. *The Lancet*, October 16, 1982, p. 876.

Rats fed either a standard diet or one supplemented with twenty-five times the RDA for vitamin A were then given a substance that induces duodenal ulcers. In the unsupplemented group, 74 percent developed ulcers, compared with 32 percent of the supplemented group. The authors suggest that vitamin A may be useful in prevention and treatment of duodenal ulcers in humans. *JPEN* 10 (January–February 1986): 74–77.

Enhanced Immunity

In a review of single nutrients and immunity, animal studies show there is an enhanced immune response when excesses of vitamin A are given; conversely, there is an increase in susceptibility to infection when there is a vitamin A deficiency. *American Journal of Clinical Nutrition* (Supplement) 35 (February 1982): 428–430.

In laboratory mice treated with cyclophosphamide and prednisolone (drugs that suppress the immune system), vitamin A supplementation restored immune response to normal level or better. *Pharmacology* 30 (April 1985): 181–187.

Note: These animal studies are very promising and indicate that scientists will investigate this connection in humans also. Up to now, most of the energy in human studies on vitamin A and immunity has been spent in relation to cancer, a very serious immune problem.

Cancer Prevention

Many studies show a correlation between high consumption of beta-carotene and/or higher vitamin A (retinol) blood levels and lowered incidence of these cancers: lung, endometrium, bronchus, bladder, breast, cervix, rectum, and the skin cancer myeloma. Such studies have been conducted all over the world including the United States, England, Finland, Japan, Norway, and Poland. What follows is a representative sampling.

In a five-year study, 8,278 Norwegian men showed a threefold decrease in lung cancer with an increase in vitamin A consumption. Beta-carotene was the major source of this vitamin. *International Journal of Cancer* 15 (1975): 561–565.

In a ten-year follow-up study of 265,118 Japanese men, the risk of lung cancer was 1.4 times greater in the men who did not eat beta-carotene-rich vegetables. *Nutrition and Cancer* 1 (1979): 67–81.

In a study conducted for nineteen years, the incidence of lung cancer among 2,107 men was inversely related to the intake of dietary beta-carotene. *Nutrition Reviews* 40 (September 1982): 265–268.

In a retrospective study in twenty-eight patients with cancer of epithelial tissues (endometrium, lung, bronchus, bladder, breast) and fifty-three patients with myeloma, a nonepithelial cancer, blood serum levels of vitamin A were lower in cancer patients than in healthy subjects, and particularly low in those with epithelial cancers. *European Journal of Cancer and Clinical Oncology* 18 (1982): 339–342.

In a study of seventy-eight women with untreated cervical cancer, blood serum values for beta-carotene, folate, and vitamin C were significantly lower than in the 240 healthy women used for controls. In addition, after cancer surgery, their beta-carotene, vitamin A, and several other nutrient levels dropped dramatically. *American Journal of Obstetrics and Gynecology* 151 (March 1, 1985): 632–635.

In a study done in England, the incidence of breast cancer was higher in women whose prediagnosis blood levels of beta-carotene (but not retinol) was lower than in the controls who did not develop cancer. *British Journal of Cancer* 49 (1984): 321–324.

After inoculating experimental mice with cancer cells, tumor metastasis (spread) was slower to appear in the group fed supplemental vitamin A. The authors conclude that vitamin A could be used to prevent metastases by keeping tumor cells confined to the encapsulated area. *Cancer Research* 45 (July 1985): 3311–3321.

In a study using hamster cells, genetic damage of the type associated with carcinogenesis was significantly reduced in the cells that were treated with vitamin A. *Journal of Clinical Investigation* 75 (June 1985): 1835–1841.

Breast cancer patients with higher blood levels of vitamin A responded twice as well to chemotherapy as women with lower levels. The authors cite Scottish researchers who report an association between improved chemotherapy response and higher vitamin A levels for patients with cancer of the breast, cancer of the bowel, and melanoma. *Medical Tribune* 23 (March 1983): 23.

Acne

In this review article, the authors point out that vitamin A has been used to treat acne since the early 1940s. In one series, one hundred patients were given 100,000 IU per day. Ninety-seven of these were "cured or almost cured." A 1981 report indicated that doses of 50,000 to 100,000 IU were ineffective, but the intake of 300,000 IU daily for three to four months was highly efficacious. The researchers postulated that the risk of toxicity at the higher dosage range was exaggerated. *Drugs* 27 (1984): 148–170.

Carotene Toxicity

In two-year studies with rats, mice, and dogs, beta-carotene was added to the diet in amounts up to 1.7 million IU per kilogram of body weight. The authors concluded that beta-carotene can be given for long periods of time virtually without risk of toxicity. *Toxicology* 36 (August 1985): 91–100.

CHAPTER 7: VITAMIN D

Overview

The author reviews what is known about the human requirement for vitamin D, the variables that influence the formation of D-3 in the skin, the symptoms of overdose, the diseases and drugs which may interfere with vitamin D metabolism, and the function of vitamin D. *Journal of the American College of Nutrition* 2 (1983): 173–199.

Intake/Synthesis/Requirements

Most patients with Crohn's disease have deficient levels of vitamin D. These patients are prone to osteomalacia and should receive vitamin D supplements. *Nutritional Review* 41:7 (1983): 213–216.

Vitamin D requirements increase with age. A total supply of 600–800 IU from all sources (food, sun, vitamin D supplements) is recommended. *American Journal of Clinical Nutrition* 36 (November 1982): 1014–1031.

In this study, healthy elderly individuals had significantly lower levels of vitamin D than did controls. The authors suggest that the elderly consider using a combination of moderate vitamin D supplementation and increased sunlight exposure to prevent subclinical vitamin D deficiency. *American Journal of Clinical Nutrition* 36 (1982): 1125–1233.

In a dietary survey of 270 healthy, highly educated, elderly people of higher-than-average income, it was found that 74 percent of the women were getting less than 75 percent of the RDA for vitamin D, and 61 percent were getting less than 50 percent. Figures for men were comparable. The authors believe that low intakes of vitamin D are of particular concern to women. *American Journal of Clinical Nutrition* 36 (August 1982): 319–331.

Osteoporosis

In this study of nineteen elderly women with and without vertebral fractures, both groups had low levels of calcium and vitamin D. After seven days of treatment with vitamin D, bloodstream levels increased in both groups, but calcium absorption increased only in women without fractures. The authors suggest that pharmacologic doses of vitamin D may be necessary to increase calcium absorption in elderly women with vertebral fractures. *Clinical Science* 66 (1984): 103–107.

Studies indicate that a combination of the two forms of D-3 may best mineralize the bone in patients with osteoporosis. Relatively lower doses of active D are required than of inactive D, which may be toxic. The authors point out that D-3 supplements may be preferable to estrogen therapy, which some physicians use to restore active D-3 concentrations, but more studies are needed. *Journal of Bone and Joint Surgery* 64-B:5 (1982): 542–560.

Cancer Prevention

The diets of nearly 2000 men were examined. During the following nineteen years, those who had the lowest intake of calcium and vitamin D had 2.7 times the risk of colorectal cancer as those with the highest intake. Other epidemiological studies have shown that exposure to sunlight and milk intake reduces the incidence of colon cancer. The authors conclude that both calcium and vitamin D may have anticancer activity. *The Lancet* I (February 9, 1985): 307–309.

Blood Pressure

In this study of over three hundred women, younger women who consumed at least 400 IU of vitamin D per day had lower systolic blood pressure. (They also had significantly higher calcium and potassium intakes.) In older women, systolic blood pressure was significantly lower in those who consumed at least the RDA of *both* calcium and vitamin D. The authors point out that this is the first report of a significant relationship between vitamin D and blood pressure, and that 50 to 75 percent of the women in the study had estimated vitamin D intakes of less than the RDA. *American Journal of Clinical Nutrition* 42 (July 1985): 135–142.

Immunity

In this small study of the blood cells of adults, vitamin D was found to affect the immune system function, with implications for treatment in some immunological diseases. *Life Sciences* 37 (July 8, 1985): 95–101.

Active vitamin D-3 plays a role in the immune-regulatory processes. *New England Journal of Medicine* 311:1 (1984): 47–49.

CHAPTER 8: VITAMIN E

Overview

This overview of the medical uses of vitamin E discusses many aspects including the advisability of supplementing diets high in PUFA with vitamin E; vitamin E as an effective antioxidant and protector against many toxic chemicals; the difficulty of detecting the subtle changes that may occur with vitamin E deficiency; and vitamin E and circulatory disease. *The New England Journal of Medicine* 308:18 (1983): 1063–1071.

Cardiovascular Disease

This entire book is devoted to vitamin E. It discusses, among other studies, those which have suggested that vitamin E might prevent deposition and accumulation of cholesterol in the arterial wall. Several other studies have suggested that vitamin E plays an important role in both lipid synthesis and degradation in the arterial wall. Results from these studies may explain the accumulation of lipids in atherosclerotic lesions. Further experiments are still in progress. *Vitamin E: Biochemical, Hematological and Clinical Aspects.* New York: Annals of the New York Academy of Sciences, vol. 393, September 30, 1982.

Rats that were fed a mixture of heated vegetable oils had enhanced platelet aggregation, when compared with rats fed unheated oils. Vitamin E in these oils, which were rich in polyunsaturated fats, was depleted 91 percent by the heat treatment. The consumption of diets rich in PUFA is generally recommended for the prevention of cardiovascular diseases; however, the use of these fats for cooking may ironically result in enhanced platelet aggregability. Provision of extra vitamin E may minimize this effect. *Lipids* 20 (July 1985): 439–448.

Aging and Cancer Prevention

Vitamin E protects vitamins A and C against oxidation; it reduces the oxidation of polyunsaturated fats and maintains the integrity of cell membranes. Corinne H. Robinson. *Normal and Therapeutic Nutrition,* 15th ed. New York: Macmillan, 1977, pp. 151–161.

Vitamin E is an effective antioxidant. In animals, it has provided protection against various toxicants including mercury, lead, benzene, and various drugs. *The New England Journal of Medicine* 308 (1983): 1063–1071.

In this study of animal cells, the authors conclude that vitamin E can minimize genetic damage associated with carcinogenesis. *Journal of Clinical Investigation* 75 (June 1985): 1835–1841.

In this study of over four hundred males, vitamin E levels in the blood were lower in the group who developed lung and colorectal cancers than in the group who did not. *Journal of the National Cancer Institute* 73 (December 1984): 1463–1468.

Low vitamin E intake may enhance the effect of selenium deficiency, which is associated with increased risk of fatal cancer. *British Medical Journal* 290 (February 9, 1985): 417–420.

In this animal study, rats were exposed to cigarette smoke. Of the group that was fed a diet deficient in vitamin E and selenium, 31 percent died. Of the group that was supplemented, only 8 percent died. The authors cite a previous study that showed that patients with lung cancer have lower vitamin E levels than healthy people. *Environmental Research* 34 (June 1984): 8–17.

In this study of over five thousand women, the risk of breast cancer was found to be 5.2 times higher for women with the lowest vitamin E levels than for those with the highest levels. *British Journal of Cancer* 49 (1984): 321–324.

The authors of this review article suggest that total fat is the most consistent dietary factor positively associated with breast cancer; PUFAs may be particularly implicated, while selenium and vitamin E are protective. *Clinical Nutrition* 4 (July–August 1985): 119–130.

The authors review the evidence relating vitamin E to breast cancer. Studies have shown that vitamin E reduces the incidence of cancer due to carcinogens. It also enhances the therapeutic effect of radiation treatment of cancer. One epidemiological study found that the group of women with the lowest blood serum vitamin E levels had five times the risk of cancer. *Journal of the American College of Nutrition* 4 (September–October 1985): 559–564.

In this study of one hundred healthy elderly people, higher levels of peroxides were found in those with lower levels of vitamins C and E. In people supplemented daily with 400 milligrams of C and/or 400 milligrams of E, peroxide levels decreased. The authors conclude that long-term supplementation of vitamins C and E can protect against free radical damage, which is thought to play a role in aging processes and degenerative diseases. *Annals of Nutrition and Metabolism* 28 (May–June 1984): 186–191.

In a study of elderly subjects, 60 percent of the patients with dementia had below-normal blood levels of vitamin E. It has been suggested that the cell damage leading to dementia may be due to free radicals. Although vitamin E deficiency is not a likely cause of dementia, it could lower the age of onset or increase the rate of progression. *The Lancet*, April 5, 1986, pp. 805–806.

Vitamin E was found to reduce the free-radical damage in experimental animals given anticancer chemotherapy. The authors conclude that this provides strong evidence for the protective use of vitamin E in cancer-free animals. They further suggest that its use during anticancer therapy is theoretically advisable because it may reduce the toxicity of some drugs, without reducing the effectiveness of the drugs. The authors cite several other studies that report the benefits of large doses of vitamin E and other antioxidant vitamins to cancer patients. *Anticancer Research* 3 (1983): 59–62.

The antioxidants alpha-tocopherol and coenzyme Q inhibited lipid peroxidation due to the chemotherapy drug Adriamycin, but did not interfere with suppression of DNA synthesis in cancer cells. *Journal of Nutrition, Science, and Vitaminology* 31 (March–April 1985): 129–137.

In this study, animals fed heated vegetable oil showed a decrease of 38–97 percent vitamin E levels in their blood and tissues. *Nutrition Reports International* 32 (November 1985): 1179–1186.

Fibrocystic Breast Disease

In a study of twenty-six women with breast disease and eight controls, 85 percent (twenty-two women) of those who received daily supplementation of 600 IU of vitamin E for eight weeks responded to the treatment. In ten women there was total disappearance of cystic lesions and breast tenderness, and in twelve women lesions decreased in number and size. The authors suggest that vitamin E supplementation may be an inexpensive and safe way of treating this disorder. *Nutrition Research* 2 (1982): 243–247.

Wound Healing

The authors note that daily doses of 800–2000 IU of vitamin E are recommended by some physicians to prevent postoperative problems in women who have undergone breast augmentation. *Plastic and Reconstructive Surgery* 69 (June 1982): 1029–1030.

Rats were fed a purified diet containing 0, 7.5, 15, 50, 200, or 1000 milligrams DL-alpha tocopherol acetate per kg of feed. The higher the dosage of vitamin E, the better the immune response, suggesting that the vitamin E requirement for optimal immune responsiveness is higher than that for other commonly used indicators of vitamin E adequacy. *Journal of Nutrition* 116 (April 1986): 675–681.

Immunity/Discoid Lupus Erythematosus

The evidence seems clear that excesses of vitamin E have an often beneficial effect on resistance to disease in a variety of experimental animals. *American Journal of Clinical Nutrition* (Supplement) 35: 431–433.

Five discoid lupus erythematosus patients given 800–2000 IU of vitamin E daily made an excellent recovery, with no side effects. This disease is normally treated with thalidomide and immunosuppressants, which have considerable side effects. The author concludes that treatment of autoimmune diseases such as DLE with vitamin E would seem preferable to the use of potentially hazardous drugs. *British Journal of Dermatology* III (July 1984): 125–126 (letter).

Seven rheumatoid arthritis patients who no longer responded to conventional therapy alone were also given 400 IU of vitamin E and 350 micrograms of selenium. In four of these patients, joint pain disappeared; in the remaining three, pain lessened and joint mobility markedly increased. *Biological Trace Element Research* 7 (May–June 1985): 195–198.

Neurological Disorders

Based on evidence from patients with disorders of fat metabolism leading to severe vitamin E deficiency, it is suggested that vitamin E is important for normal neurological function in humans. *The Lancet,* January 29, 1983, pp. 225–228.

Children with vitamin E deficiency, often due to fat malabsorption, had similar neurological disorders which respond to vitamin E therapy. *Canadian Journal of Neurological Science* 11 (November 1984): 561–564.

Other Uses

Premenstrual Syndrome: Vitamin E has been reported to improve many symptoms of PMS. *Journal of the American College of Nutrition* 3 (1984): 351–356.

Intrauterine Device Bleeding: The authors administered 100 milligrams of vitamin E every other day to fifty-one women who suffered excess menstrual bleeding after insertion of an IUD. In almost every subject, blood loss was reduced to normal. *International Journal of Fertility* 28 (1983): 55–56.

Smoking: This study found that although the levels of vitamin E in the blood of smokers and nonsmokers was similar, smokers had significantly lower levels in the cells of their lungs. Smoking seems to produce oxidant lung injury, which may play a role in the development of emphysema. Since vitamin E is an antioxidant, the authors suggest a possible role for vitamin E in the lungs' defense against cigarette smoke. *Journal of Clinical Investigation* 77 (March 1986): 789–796.

Hemodialysis-Related Anemia: Anemia is a major problem in kidney patients being treated with dialysis. In this controlled study, daily vitamin E supplementation of 600 milligrams brought about significant increases in the red blood cell count and other blood factors associated with reduction of anemia. *Nephron* 40 (August 1985): 440–445.

Kidney Disease: Sixteen children with hemolytic uremic syndrome were treated with vitamin E: 94 percent recovered completely compared to 36–50 percent of patients previously treated with other therapies. *Archives of Disorders in Children* 59 (May 1984): 401–404.

CHAPTER 9: VITAMIN K

Osteoporosis

Blood levels of vitamin K in patients with osteoporosis were approximately one third the level of those in an apparently healthy control group. The authors conclude that low levels of the vitamin may be a factor in the development of osteoporosis. *Journal of Clinical Endocrinology and Metabolism* 60 (June 1985): 1268–1269.

Behavior

Vitamin K–deficient animals became less active and suffered from general malaise. These results suggest that vitamin K deficiency may contribute to physical and psychiatric symptoms. *Physiology and Behavior* 34 (May 1985): 727–734.

CHAPTER 11: VITAMIN B-1 (Thiamin)

Surgery

Elderly patients experienced a significant lowering of thiamin levels in the blood after surgery. The authors suggest that thiamin deficiency may be one factor in postoperative mental confusion and overall deterioration in this population, and that more attention should be paid to assessing their thiamin status. *Age and Ageing* 11 (1982): 101–107.

Thiamin Intake and Absorption

Severe disease increasingly interferes with the dietary intake of thiamin, and alcoholism interferes with the absorption of thiamin in a major fashion. *American Journal of Clinical Nutrition* 36 (November 1982): 1067–1082.

Immunity

In this study, thiamin-deficient experimental animals showed less response to immunization vaccinations. *Proceedings of the Society of Experimental Biology and Medicine* 77 (1951): 526–530.

Psychiatric Disease

In a study of psychiatric patients, schizophrenics and alcoholics as a group were significantly overrepresented in patients who were low in thiamin. *British Journal of Psychiatry* 141 (1982): 271.

A survey of 172 unselected psychiatric patients showed 30 percent to be biochemically deficient in thiamin; only 1 of these had clinical symptoms of deficiency. Inadequate intake of vitamins, particularly B-1, can result in mental illness. *Clinical Neuropharmacology* 8 (July–September 1985): 286–293.

Cancer

The authors speculate that thiamin supplementation (in this study, 100 milligrams per day) could help prevent cell damage, fibrinogenesis, and collagen breakdown in cancer patients. *Journal of Nutrition, Growth and Cancer* 1 (July–December 1984): 207–210.

Toxicity

Toxicity of thiamin was only seen in doses thousands of times larger than normal. There have been no toxic effects of thiamin administered by mouth reported in humans. Robert S. Goodhart and Maurice E. Shils. *Modern Nutrition in Health and Disease*, 6th ed. Philadelphia: Lea and Febiger, 1980.

CHAPTER 12: VITAMIN B-2 (Riboflavin)

Cataracts

A study in laboratory rats showed that a diet deficient in vitamin B-2 causes cataracts in from two to three months. Other changes in the eye also occurred. *American Journal of Ophthalmology* 14 (1931): 1005–1009.

Riboflavin deficiency has been linked to cataract formation in some studies. Low riboflavin intake or impaired riboflavin utilization could lead to an increase in cataract formation. *American Journal of Clinical Nutrition* 34 (May 1981): 861–863.

In an experiment with rats, the results indicate that vitamin B-2 is fairly active in maintaining transparency of the lens of the eye. *International Journal for Vitamin and Nutrition Research* 53 (1983): 243–250.

Exercise

Riboflavin plays a role in energy production. The daily allowance for riboflavin is proportional to energy needs. Regular exercise has been shown to increase the daily needs of riboflavin. Mild deficiencies have been shown in athletes undergoing strenuous daily exercise. *Nutrition Research* 4 (1984): 201–208.

Weight-reducing women require more than the RDA of riboflavin during periods of nonexercise and exercise. *American Journal of Clinical Nutrition* 41 (February 1985): 270–277.

Nervous Symptoms

In a study of psychiatric patients, 53 percent were deficient in at least one of these vitamins: thiamin, riboflavin, and vitamin B-6. The authors conclude that a deficiency in one or several of these nutrients has a primary role in the cause of emotional disorder. *British Journal of Psychiatry* 141 (1982): 271–272.

Carpal Tunnel Syndrome

A man with carpal tunnel syndrome was given 50 milligrams riboflavin and 500 milligrams pyridoxine (B-6) daily for a total of eight months. All his CTS symptoms disappeared. *Proceedings of the National Academy of Science* 81 (November 1984): 7076–7078.

Sickle Cell Anemia

This study of sickle cell anemia patients suggests that nearly half were deficient in vitamin B-2. *American Journal of Clinical Nutrition* 38 (December 1983): 884–887.

Esophageal Cancer

In this animal study, nearly half the subjects fed a riboflavin-free diet developed precancerous or cancerous tumors of the esophagus. The authors conclude that riboflavin helps to maintain the lining of the mouth and esophagus, and its deficiency may increase the susceptibility of these tissues to carcinogens. *Journal of the National Cancer Institute* 72 (April 1984): 941–948.

Anemia

Riboflavin given with iron enhanced the recovery of microcytic anemia in men and children. *Human Nutrition. Clinical Nutrition* 37C (1983): 413–425.

Oral Contraceptives

In this study, riboflavin deficiency was found to be more prevalent in women taking oral contraceptives than in women who were not. *American Journal of Clinical Nutrition* 35 (March 1982): 495–501.

Immunity

Riboflavin deficiency in animals results in a diminished ability to produce antibodies in response to test antigens. *American Journal of Clinical Nutrition* (Supplement) 35 (February 1982): 421.

Detecting and Alleviating Deficiencies

In an Indian study, 4 milligrams of riboflavin (the RDA) failed to correct deficiencies in half the subjects. *Nutrition Research* 2 (1982): 147–153.

The authors studied forty-two adolescent boys with no clinical symptoms of riboflavin deficiency, but biochemical testing showed that 38 percent were deficient. *American Journal of Clinical Nutrition* 39 (May 1984): 787–791.

CHAPTER 13: VITAMIN B-3 (Niacin and Niacinamide)

Blood Lipids—Cholesterol and Triglycerides

Both cholesterol and triglycerides may be lowered 50 percent or more by niacin therapy. The authors believe that niacin is the agent of choice in many patients with hyperlipidemia. *Drug Therapy*, August 1984, pp. 62–70.

Niacin was given in a time-release or unmodified form to patients with elevated triglyceride and/or LDL cholesterol levels. The unmodified form was a more effective therapy and resulted in fewer side effects than the time-release niacin. Triglycerides were decreased by 42 percent (vs. 1 percent), LDL cholesterol decreased 30 percent (vs. 25 percent), and HDL cholesterol increased 22 percent (vs. 9 percent). *Metabolism* 34 (July 1985): 642–650.

When niacin (3 grams per day) and clofibrate were compared, niacin was from 28 to 48 percent more effective in lowering cholesterol and triglycerides in the blood. Niacin also created a more desirable HDL/LDL ratio. *Atherosclerosis* 51 (1984): 251–259.

A previously untreated diabetic was treated with insulin and diet. His triglyceride level dropped from 258 to 158; this was sharply reduced further when niacin therapy was added. Other studies have shown that triglyceride levels can be lowered by more than 60 percent by nicotinic acid. *Postgraduate Medicine Journal* 57 (August 1981): 511–515.

Cancer Prevention

In this animal study, only 14 percent of the subjects that were given niacinamide along with a potent carcinogen developed pancreatic cancer, as compared with 43 percent of those that were given the carcinogen alone. The authors conclude from this and previous research that niacinamide inhibits cancer at several sites, and that since niacin has low toxicity, it may be useful in cancer prevention. *Journal of the National Cancer Institute* 73 (September 1984): 767–770.

In mice with laboratory-induced breast cancer, the effectiveness of radiation therapy with or without the administration of niacin was assessed. The average size of the tumor in mice given niacinamide with radiation was decreased by 86 percent two weeks after treatment, and remained 79 percent lower after four weeks. The authors suggest that niacin sensitizes tissue to the effects of radiation and may have a role in the treatment of malignant tumors. *Cancer Research* 45 (August 1985): 3609–3614.

190   Design Your Own Vitamin and Mineral Program

Epilepsy

The authors discuss their study and previous studies which show that nicotinamide (as well as vitamins E and B-6 and calcium pantothenate) may be useful in the treatment of epilepsy together with anticonvulsants. They suggest that such combined treatment would not only give an anticonvulsant effect, but could also improve the nutrition and structural metabolism of the brain, a matter of great importance. *Byolleten Eksperimental noi Biologii i Meditsiny* 94(9): 61–64.

CHAPTER 14: VITAMIN B-6 (Pyridoxine)

Overview

A deficiency in vitamin B-6 results in skin and nervous system disorders, kidney disorders, depression of immune responses, anemia, and carpal tunnel syndrome. Studies have shown deficiencies and/or an increased need for B-6 in oral contraceptive users, alcoholics, during certain situations such as exposure to radiation, certain drugs, cardiac failure, pregnancy, and lactation. *American Journal of Medical Technology* 49:1 (1983): 17–21.

Bioavailability

The authors studied the bioavailability of B-6 from several foods and found that the amount of B-6 in foods does not necessarily represent the amount of the vitamin available to humans. In fact, the bioavailability of B-6 from natural sources is limited. *Journal of Nutrition* 113 (1983): 2412–2420.

Emotional Illness

Of the psychiatric patients admitted to the hospital in this study, 53 percent were deficient in at least one of the following: B-6, thiamin, and riboflavin. B-6 is associated with depression and other emotional disorders and the authors suggest that along with riboflavin, B-6 deficiency has a primary role in the cause of emotional disorder. *British Journal of Psychiatry* 141 (1982): 271–272.

The authors conclude that the current data suggest that as many as 20 percent of a medically cleared population of outpatient depressives may suffer from a B-6 deficit. They point out that nutrition, diet, and vitamin levels have received very little attention in the psychiatric literature, and implicate reducing diets as playing a possible role in depression. *Biological Psychiatry* 9:4 (1984): 613–616.

In this study of eleven psychiatric patients, 57–100 percent of the depressed patients and 25–50 percent of the obsessive-compulsive patients had inadequate levels of B-6. The authors ask, "Does depressive illness cause vitamin B-6 inadequacy, or vice-versa?" *Nutrition Reports International* 27 (April 1983): 867–873.

The authors describe how 500 milligrams of B-6 were effective in treating an acutely schizophrenic patient who did not respond to other psychotropic medications. They recommend that B-6 be considered as an alternative treatment for this disorder. *Biological Psychiatry* 18:11 (1983): 1321–1328.

Carpal Tunnel Syndrome

A patient with carpal tunnel syndrome (CTS) who was given 500-milligram B-6 and 50-milligram riboflavin supplements experienced complete disappearance of his symptoms. *Proceedings of the National Academy of Sciences* 81 (November 1984): 7076–7078.

In this small study, four out of six CTS patients claimed some partial relief after B-6 supplementation. The authors note that a number of recent studies report that patients with CTS respond to pyridoxine treatment, but that a large double-blind controlled study is necessary to fully test the efficacy of this treatment. *Annals of Neurology* 15 (January 1984): 104–107.

Childhood Epilepsy and Autism

Pyridoxine-dependent seizures (PDS) in infants, which should be suspected in every infant with convulsions before eighteen months of age, were controlled by administration of B-6. Failure to treat PDS with B-6 promptly results in severe mental retardation or death. *Annals of Neurology* 17 (February 1985): 117–120.

Many forms of infant and childhood epilepsy respond to B-6 treatment. All infants with refractory epileptic seizure must be given an adequate trial of B-6. *Archives of Disease in Childhood* 58 (1983): 1034–1036 (letter).

The effects of vitamin B-6 and magnesium supplementation on sixty autistic children were examined in a double-blind trial. The combination resulted in a significant improvement in many aspects of autistic behavior. *Biological Psychiatry* 20 (May 1985): 467–478.

Premenstrual Syndrome

The researchers report overwhelming evidence in both their study and in others that 100 milligrams per day of B-6 appears to have a 60 to 80 percent success rate in the treatment of PMS. B-6 has been effective in cases where progesterone has failed; owing to the low toxicity of B-6, it is the authors' opinion that it should be tried as the first line of treatment in PMS. *The Practitioner* 228 (April 1984): 425–427.

Pregnancy and Breastfeeding

During the last month of their pregnancy, the women in this study were shown to have consumed an average of only 50 percent of the RDA for B-6. For breastfeeding women, intake rose after delivery, but only to 60 percent of the RDA. *Journal of the American Dietetic Association* 84 (November 1984): 1339–1344.

In a study of twenty-four mothers and their infants, only those who received supplements of 10–20 milligrams of B-6 daily produced milk which met the American Academy of Pediatrics recommended concentration of B-6. *American Journal of Clinical Nutrition* 41 (January 1985): 21–31.

In this double-blind trial, 52 pregnant women were given pyridoxine supplements. Those who received 7.5 to 20 milligrams per day delivered babies whose Apgar scores were significantly higher than the infants of mothers who received 2.6 milligrams. *Journal of Nutrition* 114 (May 1984): 977–988.

Cardiovascular Disease

Based on the results of this controlled study of men with heart disease, the authors conclude that vitamin B-6 deficiency may influence vascular connective tissue and thrombogenesis (clotting). *Atherosclerosis* 55 (June 1985): 357–361.

Experiments giving animals diets deficient in vitamin B-6 have resulted in an enhanced risk of cardiovascular disease in the subjects, and other experiments suggest the same may be true for humans. The authors also point out that exposure to environmental pollution causes vitamin B-6 deficiency. *Medical Hypotheses* 15 (December 1984): 361–367.

Immunity

In this overview, the authors point out that pyridoxine deficiencies cause more profound effects on immune system functions than deficiencies of any other B vitamin. Both human and animal studies have shown B-6 to be involved in a wide variety of organs and processes of the immune system. *American Journal of Clinical Nutrition* (Supplement) 35 (February 1982): 418–421.

In laboratory animals, vitamin B-6 deficiency impaired the immune response and increased the animals' susceptibility to a cancer-causing virus. *Journal of Nutrition* 114 (May 1984): 938–945.

In a study on humans who were undergoing hemodialysis, B-6 levels were low and the immune system was impaired in over half the subjects. After they were given B-6 supplements, their immune systems were improved. *Nephron* 38 (September 1984): 9–16.

Kidney Disease

In a study of humans with kidney disease, the average level of B-6 in the blood was significantly lower than in the controls. The authors conclude that the development of immune dysfunction and cardiovascular disease in patients with kidney disease may be related to B-6 deficiency. *International Journal of Vitamin Research* 54 (October–December 1984): 313–319.

The administration of 25–200 milligrams of B-6 daily led to decreased oxalate secretion in patients with a form of hereditary kidney disorder. (Excess oxalate may lead to calcium deposits in the kidney, which may in turn lead to kidney failure and death.) *New England Journal of Medicine* 312 (April 11, 1985): 953–957.

In a group of twenty-two patients with oxalate kidney stones, a dosage of 250–500 milligrams of B-6 was found to be an effective treatment. *Canadian Medical Association Journal* 131 (July 1984): 14.

Based on his experience with a patient to whom he gave 500 milligrams of pyridoxine a day for seventeen months, the author of this letter suggests that pyridoxine therapy can reverse the course of renal failure in certain infants. *New England Journal of Medicine* 311 (September 20, 1984): 798–799.

Asthma

In this study, fifteen adult asthmatics had significantly lower pyridoxal levels than did sixteen healthy controls. Those subjects who took 50 milligrams of B-6 daily reported a dramatic decrease in the frequency and severity of wheezing or asthmatic attacks while taking the supplement. *American Journal of Clinical Nutrition* 41 (1985): 684–688.

Sickle Cell Anemia

Sixteen patients with sickle cell anemia had pyridoxal levels significantly lower than sixteen healthy controls. B-6 has been shown to have anti-sickling properties, and these studies suggest that pyridoxine supplementation may have therapeutic benefit. *American Journal of Clinical Nutrition* 40 (August 1984): 235–239.

Diabetes

According to the author of this letter, one quarter of the adult diabetic patients have below-normal levels of pyridoxine. Diabetics may not metabolize B-6 normally and may need more than the RDA. Further research seems to be indicated. *American Journal of Clinical Nutrition* 39 (May 1984): 841–842.

Chinese Restaurant Syndrome

This study shows that the symptoms of Chinese Restaurant Syndrome caused by monosodium glutamate sensitivity fail to recur after treatment with 50–200 milligrams of pyridoxine. *Hoppe-Seyler's Zeitschrift fur Physiologishe Chemie* 365:3 (1984): 405–414.

Melanoma

In animal experiments, topical injections of B-6 retarded the growth of malignant melanoma. In one study, the tumors of the treated mice weighed 62 percent less than in untreated controls; in another, tumor growth was inhibited by 39 percent. *Nutrition and Cancer* 7 (January–June 1985): 43–52.

Toxicity

The authors report seven cases of neurotoxicity resulting from massive intakes (2 to 6 grams per day) of B-6. Symptoms of toxicity include unsteady gait, numb feet, numbness and clumsiness of the hands. In most of the cases, B-6 was the only nutritional supplement used by the patient. All patients improved substantially following withdrawal of B-6. *New England Journal of Medicine* 309 (August 25, 1983): 445–448.

In this study, a group of twenty-two patients received a dosage of 250–500 milligrams of pyridoxine with no ill effects, and the authors conclude that these amounts are safe for long periods (up to six years). *Canadian Medical Association Journal* 131 (July 1984): 14.

CHAPTER 15: VITAMIN B-12 (Cobalamin)

Psychiatric Disorders

The authors of this review recommend that the patient who fails to respond to treatment of any psychiatric symptom complex should be evaluated for B-12 deficiency. *Biological Psychiatry* 16 (1981): 197–205.

Patients who do not have severe anemia may develop neurologic abnormalities before the underlying vitamin B-12 deficiency is recognized. *Annals of Family Practice* 25 (January 1982): 111–115.

In one study, over 73 percent of aged patients with organic psychiatric disorders had low blood levels of B-12; in another study of aged patients with mental disorders, 55 percent and 25 percent had low B-12 levels. B-12 deficiency has been shown to be significantly more frequent in patients with Alzheimer-type dementia than in others. The authors point out that the clarification of this observation may provide an important clue in our understanding of this disease, since prolonged low B-12 levels may produce permanent neurological changes in these patients. *Age and Ageing* 13 (1984): 101–105.

Fatigue

In a double-blind study, twenty-eight patients complaining of fatigue were given injections of B-12 or a placebo for four weeks. The group that received the placebo for the first two weeks and then B-12 for the next two weeks showed a favorable response with respect to general well-being and happiness only when they were given the B-12. The group that received the B-12 for the first two weeks and placebo for the next two weeks did not notice any difference between the active and the placebo treatment. This suggests that the effects of B-12 may persist for a period of at least four weeks. *Journal of Nutrition* 30 (1973): 277–279.

Cancer Prevention

In this animal study, mice were implanted with tumor cells. Only two of the fifty that received B-12 and ascorbic acid developed tumors; all fifty of the untreated mice developed tumors. Vitamin B-12 and vitamin C given separately in the same doses did not have the same effect. *IRCS Medical Science* 12 (September 1984): 813.

Nitrous Oxide

Prolonged excess exposure to nitrous oxide may result in B-12 anemia. *Journal of Clinical Pathology* 33 (1980): 909–916.

CHAPTER 16: FOLIC ACID

Depression

Folic acid deficiency has been suggested as a cause of depression. *Psychosomatics* 21 (1980): 926–929.

In this study, folic acid blood levels were significantly lower in the depressed patients, leading the authors to conclude that a folic acid deficiency depression may exist. *Psychosomatics* 21 (November 1980): 926–929.

In this review article, the authors point out that depression is a common manifestation of severe folate deficiency. Depressed patients with folate deficiency had more severe illness and responded less well to conventional antidepressant therapy than those without this deficiency. In addition, those in whom the deficiency was treated made better recoveries than those with untreated folate deficiency. *Lancet* II (July 28, 1984): 196–198.

Mental Retardation

Large doses of folic acid (2 milligrams three times a day) have been reported to improve the behavior of adults with a chromosomal abnormality linked with mental retardation. Female carriers of the syndrome, who are apt to be mildly retarded, might also benefit from folate supplementation. *American Journal of Medicine* 77 (October 1984): 602–611.

Immunity

This overview cites studies indicating that deficiencies of folic acid lead to a reduction in the resistance to disease in humans and animals. Both antibody and white cell production are affected. *American Journal of Clinical Nutrition* (Supplement) 35 (February 1982): 421.

Pregnancy and Birth Defects

Mothers of children born with harelip received 10 milligrams of folic acid plus a multivitamin daily prior to or during the first trimester of their subsequent pregnancies. Only one of the supplemented mothers gave birth to another child with harelip; fifteen of the unsupplemented group had children with this birth defect. The authors state that the results are highly suggestive that moderate supplementation may reduce the rate of recurrence of some birth defects. *The Lancet,* July 24, 1982: 217.

Pregnant guinea pigs were fed either an RDA-sufficient diet alone or one with folic acid and vitamin C supplements. In the unsupplemented group, 68.8 percent of the fetuses did not survive to midpregnancy, compared with 17.5 percent in the supplemented group. The authors conclude that during early pregnancy intakes of these two nutrients well above the RDA may be needed for optimal reproductive performance in humans. *British Journal of Nutrition* 55 (January–February 1986): 23–35.

Oral Contraceptives and Cervical Dysplasia

Oral contraceptives may cause localized rather than systemic folate deficiency, which could alter the susceptibility of cervical cells to cancer-causing substances. In this controlled study of oral contraceptive users with mild to moderate cervical dysplasia, the women who were supplemented with 10 milligrams folic acid daily showed significant improvement over those who were unsupplemented. The authors conclude that localized changes in folate metabolism may be misdiagnosed as cervical dysplasia, or that these changes are an integral part of the condition and that dysplasia may be arrested or reversed with folic acid supplementation. *American Journal of Clinical Nutrition* 35 (1982): 73–82.

The author cites studies that suggest that folic acid supplementation may help reduce the risk of cervical cancer in women taking combination oral contraceptives. One study involved eighty-nine women with mild to moderate cervical neoplasia who had been taking combination oral contraceptives for six months or longer. This double-blind random study concluded that folate (10 milligrams per day for three months) had a substantial benefit on cervical epithelium. There was no change among the women in the placebo group. *Journal of the American Medical Association* 244:7 (1980): 633–634.

Oral contraceptives impair folate metabolism. In this study, the mean blood level of folate in women using the Pill decreased, and it required up to three months for them to return to normal after the Pill was stopped. *CMA Journal* 126 (February 1, 1982): 244–247.

Impaired Absorption and Metabolism of Folic Acid

Anticonvulsants and sulfasalazine (prescribed for inflammatory bowel disease) may interfere with folate absorption. Gastric surgery and intestinal conditions can also interfere. There is some evidence that the physiological process of aging influences the intestinal absorption of folate. *American Journal of Clinical Nutrition* 36 (November 1982): 1060–1066.

In this study, blood levels of folate in a healthy woman fell by 29 percent when she received therapeutic doses of aspirin. (However, the authors point out that it is not known whether tissue stores were affected.) *Journal of Laboratory and Clinical Medicine* 103 (June 1984): 944–948.

In animal studies it has been shown that folic acid is lost from the liver when nitrous oxide is administered as an anesthetic gas. *American Journal of Clinical Nutrition* 34 (1981): 2412–2417.

Adverse Effects

Oral supplementation of folic acid lowers the plasma zinc levels and increases zinc excretion. Therefore women with cervical dysplasia undergoing folic acid treatment may be particularly prone to zinc deficiency; this may be a hazard especially in users of oral contraceptives because this medication may also lower zinc levels. *Journal of the National Cancer Institute* 74 (January 1985): 263 (letter).

CHAPTER 17: PANTOTHENIC ACID

Immunity

In human and animal studies, pantothenic acid deficiencies depress antibody responsiveness to antigens. *American Journal of Clinical Nutrition* (Supplement) 35 (February 1982): 421.

Physical Stress and Exercise

In this overview, the authors discuss why pantothenic acid has long been considered an antistress vitamin. They cite several studies of pantothenic supplementation, including: laboratory rats who showed a significant improvement in exercise tolerance and resistance to radiation-induced injury; humans who better withstood cold water stress; and the delay in the onset of fatigue. *Journal of Sports Medicine* 24 (1984): 26–29.

Wound Healing and Physical Injury

Experimental animals who were given pantothenic acid supplements before and after surgery healed better than those who were unsupplemented. The authors conclude that such supplementation appears to have a beneficial effect on wound healing. *American Journal of Clinical Nutrition* 41 (March 1985): 578–589.

A drug combination containing a form of pantothenic acid was applied to animals before and after exposure to UV radiation. As a result, they experienced less skin inflammation and more rapid healing of skin inflammation. *Arzneimittelforshung* 32 (1982): 1096–1100.

A drug combination containing a form of pantothenic acid was applied to students with sports injuries. They experienced decreased swelling and increased joint mobility. *Arzneimittelforshung* 33 (1983): 792–795.

Rheumatoid Arthritis

In this overview, the authors point out that lower blood levels of pantothenic acid are associated with arthritis. They cite studies that show that pantothenic acid supplements have helped alleviate symptoms of this disease, and urge that further trials are indicated. *The Practitioner* 224 (February 1980): 208–211.

Nervous System

The authors point out that homopantothenic acid (HOPA), a naturally occurring substance, is now in widespread clinical use as a potent agent to improve epilepsy, postencephalitic sequelae, mental retardation, and mental and physical disorders in children. *Tohoku Journal of Experimental Medicine* 140 (1983): 45–51.

CHAPTER 18: BIOTIN

In this study, eight patients experienced marked improvement in their hemodialysis-related neurologic disorders with daily supplementation of 10 milligrams of biotin. The authors conclude that biotin supplementation is effective in preventing and treating the neurological disorders that can result from chronic hemodialysis. They recommend that biotin therapy be started in patients with advanced renal failure before severe symptoms appear. *Nephron* 36 (1984): 183–186.

Dermatitis

Treatment of the mothers of breast-fed infants with seborrheic dermatitis by injection of pharmacologic doses of biotin has been reported to be of benefit. *Nutrition in Health and Disease*, sixth ed. Philadelphia: Lea and Febiger, 1980, pp. 274–279.

CHAPTER 19: CHOLINE, INOSITOL, AND PABA

Atherosclerosis

Nine men and nine women with high triglycerides and cholesterol were given lecithin. Triglycerides, cholesterol, and platelet aggregation were all significantly decreased, and HDL cholesterol was increased. The authors conclude that lecithin may be a useful adjunct in the treatment of atherosclerosis. *Biochemical and Medical Metabolism and Biology* 35 (January–February 1986): 31–39.

CHAPTER 20: VITAMIN C

Tissue Repair and Wound Healing

In this review article, the authors conclude that clinical studies provide evidence that wound healing in subjects judged not deficient in vitamin C can be significantly accelerated with supplements in daily dosages of 500 to 3000 milligrams. The subjects of the studies reviewed included those recovering from surgery, other injuries, pressure sores, and leg ulcers. *Oral Surgery*, March 1982: 231–236.

Antioxidant

In a study of one hundred elderly people, in those who were supplemented with 400 milligrams of vitamin C and/or 200 milligrams of vitamin E, serum lipid peroxides declined to as little as 74 percent of initial levels, after one year. The authors conclude that long-term supplementation of moderate amounts of these nutrients presumably protects against free radical damage, which may play a role in aging and the development of degenerative diseases. *Annals of Nutrition and Metabolism* 28 (May–June 1984): 186–191.

Immunity

Vitamin C has been shown to reduce symptoms experienced by asthmatics challenged with histamine, or methacholine. Vitamin C significantly reduced airway reactivity to methacholine aerosol. *American Review of Respiratory Disease* 127 (February 1983): 143–147.

In a study of forty-four pairs of twins living apart, there was an apparent protective effect of vitamin C. Among these pairs the vitamin C group got 19 percent fewer colds, the total duration was 38 percent less, total severity was 22 percent less, and intensity was 20 percent less than in the placebo group. *Acta Geneticae Medicae et Gemollologiae* 30 (1981): 249–255.

Vitamin C levels in serum and body tissues lower with age. Vitamin C enhanced the immune responsiveness in subjects who received doses of 500 milligrams. The authors conclude that vitamin C should be considered as a possibly successful nontoxic and inexpensive substance which may have some application in improving immune competence of the aging. *Gerontology* 29 (1983): 305–310.

Cancer Prevention

Vitamin C has been shown to be effective in blocking the formation of nitrosamines and similar compounds. The author of this review article evaluates studies that give evidence of vitamin C's role in preventing bladder cancer, stomach cancer, colon cancer, cervical and uterine cancer, and esophageal and lung cancer. There are specific cases such as recurrent bladder cancer or achlorhydria (low stomach acid) in which vitamin C may prove useful at high doses. *Seminars in Oncology* 10 (September 1983): 294–298.

In a study of 78 women with cervical cancer, blood levels for vitamin C, beta-carotene, and folate were significantly lower than the 240 healthy women used for controls. *American Journal of Obstetrics and Gynecology* 151 (March 1, 1985): 632–635.

In this animal study, a mixture of vitamins C and B-12 was given to mice implanted with tumor cells. All fifty of the unsupplemented mice developed tumors, but only two of the fifty supplemented mice had tumors; these tumors were smaller than those in the controls. *IRCS Medical Science* 12 (September 1984): 813.

In one study, one hundred advanced cancer patients who received large supplemental doses of ascorbic acid lived from 4.2 to 20 times longer than the controls. The authors conclude that ascorbic acid is of definite value in the treatment of patients with advanced cancer. *Proceedings of the National Academy of Sciences* 73:10 (October 1976): 3685–3689.

Smoking

Smoking cigarettes raises the requirement for vitamin C. *American Journal of Clinical Nutrition* 34 (1981): 1347–1355.

This study of smokers revealed that they had lower bloodstream levels of vitamin C than nonsmokers. Two to four times as many smokers as nonsmokers had vitamin C deficiencies in the near-scurvy range. Smokers have a special need for vitamin C, and a normal dietary intake may not adequately keep their vitamin C level within a normal range. *Federation Proceedings* 43 (1984): 861.

Increases in blood pressure immediately following cigarette smoking were lowered by 400 milligrams of vitamin C. *Nutrition Research* 3 (1983): 653–661.

Oral Contraceptives

Women taking long-term oral contraceptives eliminate vitamin C from their bodies at a higher rate. They may need increased daily doses of vitamin C. In addition, vitamin C has been shown to enhance the levels of certain hormones in the blood (estradiol) and it is possible that the dosage of estrogen in the Pill may be reduced with vitamin C supplementation. *Annals of Nutrition and Metabolism* 28 (May–June 1984): 186–191.

Coronary Heart Disease

In this review article, the author discusses studies of the beneficial effects of vitamin C on veins and arteries. In one study, the deep vein thrombosis rate was lowered by 50 percent in surgical patients given 1000 milligrams of vitamin C daily. In another clinical trial, atherosclerotic patients given vitamin C could walk farther without feeling pain or breathlessness. Vitamin C may help to prevent cholestrol deposits by preventing and repairing damaged arterial walls and mobilizing cholesterol away from the arterial wall to the liver. The author suggests that atherosclerosis is a long-term deficiency of Vitamin C. *American Heart Journal* 88:3 (1974): 387–388.

High intakes of vitamin C or of fruits and green vegetables which are high in vitamin C have been related to lowered mortality from stroke and heart disease. The author suggests that ascorbic acid has a preventive effect on hypertension. *International Journal for Vitamin and Nutrition Research* 54 (1984): 343–347.

Two studies show that when people with high cholesterol were given 300–1000 milligrams of vitamin C daily, their cholesterol levels dropped. *The Lancet*, October 20, 1984: 907.

Correlations between serum HDL cholesterol and vitamin C intake were positive and significant in women. In men, high levels of HDLs seem to be associated with very high vitamin C intakes. If an adequate supply of vitamin C is necessary for the maintenance of optimal HDL levels, then perhaps the requirements of men are substantially higher than those of women. *American Journal of Clinical Nutrition* 40 (December 1984): 1334–1338.

Optimum Vitamin C Intake

The author arrived at an estimated body pool of vitamin C of 5000 milligrams for a 70-kilogram person. An intake of 200 milligrams daily would maintain this level. This refers to people who are free from stress. Individuals who have high levels of physical activity, pregnancy, mental stress, diabetes, injury, infection, cancer, atherosclerosis, pollution, and medications may require much higher dosages. *Nutrition and Health* 1 (1981): 66–77.

Human beings are genetically programmed to consume the diet available to our ancient hunter-gatherer ancestors, who evolved forty thousand years ago. The authors estimate that these people consumed a diet containing almost 400 milligrams of vitamin C each day. *The New England Journal of Medicine* 312 (January 31, 1985): 283–289.

In a study of adolescent boys, the group that was given 70 milligrams of vitamin C daily improved their aerobic work capacity by 10 percent. The authors conclude that the optimal intake of vitamin C is about 80–100 milligrams a day. *International Journal for Vitamin and Nutrition Research* 54 (January–March 1984): 55–60.

Rats maintain a body pool of vitamin C five times greater than the pool calculated for humans. *Journal of Biological Chemistry* 230 (1958): 923.

The author reviews data concerning synthesis of vitamin C in animals and ingestion of vitamin C in non–vitamin C–producing animals, both under normal conditions and under stress. He concludes that these data suggest that the optimum daily intake of vitamin C for humans is between 250 and 4000 milligrams. *Proceedings of the National Academy of Sciences* 71:11 (1974): 4442–4446.

The author notes that most animals produce their own vitamin C, at the rate of up to 275 milligrams per kilogram daily, and this is much higher than the RDA for humans, which is .9 milligrams per kilogram. In animals that must obtain vitamin C from the diet, about ten times this amount, necessary to prevent scurvy, was needed to maintain health, and up to 40 milligrams per kilogram was needed to survive the stresses of long-term captivity. Research suggests that the amount of vitamin C necessary to prevent scurvy is less than that required for maximal enzyme activity. *The New England Journal of Medicine* 314 (April 3, 1986): 892–902.

Toxicity and Adverse Effects

Based on two studies in which adults were supplemented with 3000–10,000 milligrams of vitamin C daily, the authors conclude that the probability of oxalate stone formation due to ingestion of vitamin C is very small. *International Journal for Vitamin and Nutrition Research* 54 (April–September 1984): 245–249.

In a two-year toxicity study, experimental mice and rats were given very high doses of ascorbic acid (up to 2800 and 13,800 milligrams per kilogram of body weight, respectively). No evidence of toxicity was found. *Journal of Toxicology and Environmental Health* 14 (October 1984): 605–609.

Previous studies have suggested that high doses of vitamin C destroy B-12 in the body. More recent studies, using superior techniques, have shown no significant evidence of destruction of B-12 body stores with up to 2000 milligrams of vitamin C. *Scottish Medical Journal* 27 (1982): 240–243.

Other Uses

Birth Defects: Neural tube defects (spina bifida, anencephalus) are associated with low levels of vitamin C and folic acid. *Canadian Medical Association Journal* 129 (November 15, 1983): 1088–1091.

When rats were fed a high-sugar diet designed to cause cataracts, only 6 percent of the group supplemented with vitamin C developed cataracts, versus 69 percent of the unsupplemented control group. When the sugar was removed from the diets, all of those rats started on vitamin-C supplementation lost their cataracts, versus 67 percent of those who were unsupplemented. Even though rats synthesize their own vitamin C, supplementation delayed the progression of these cataracts and hastened their regression. *Nutrition Report International* 33 (April 1986): 665–668.

Pregnancy Complications: In a study of eighty-seven pregnant women, 74 percent of those with abruptio placentae had significantly lower blood levels of vitamin C than those without this complication. The authors conclude that a deficiency of vitamin C could result in symptoms observed in this complication of pregnancy. *Human Nutrition and Clinical Nutrition* 39C (May–June 1985): 233–238.

Male Infertility: Infertile men with lowered sperm count were given 1000 milligrams of vitamin C daily. Throughout the several weeks of the study, there was a continuous rise in the percentage of normal sperm, sperm viability, and sperm motility. *Journal of the American Medical Association* 249 (May 27, 1983): 2747–2748.

Depression and Mania: In two studies, patients improved when treated with a low-vanadium diet or high doses of ascorbic acid. *Nutritional Review* 40:10 (October 1982): 293–295.

AIDS: Taking vitamin C to bowel tolerance (40–100 grams daily) is reported to put AIDS (Acquired Immune Deficiency Syndrome) into extended clinical remission. The author recommends all at risk for AIDS to take vitamin C to bowel tolerance. *Mental Hypothesis* 14 (August 1984): 423–433.

The Elderly: Vitamin C therapy of 1000 milligrams per day given to institutionalized elderly led to an improvement of their nutritional state and a reduction in petechial hemorrhages (pin-sized red dots under the skin). *American Journal of Clinical Nutrition* 34 (1981): 871–876.

Hospital Patients: The vitamin C levels of 199 elderly hospital patients were measured upon admission. Those with low vitamin C levels had a mortality rate of 45 percent during the study, but only 27 percent of those with higher vitamin C levels died, although the severity of illness was the same in both groups. In addition, half were given 200 milligrams of vitamin C daily; half were given a placebo. Those with low initial levels of vitamin C who received the supplement tended to improve more than those given the placebo. The authors conclude that supplementation of patients who have low vitamin C levels may improve their prognosis. *International Journal for Vitamin and Nutrition Research* 54 (January–March 1984): 65–74.

Drug Hepatotoxicity: In laboratory mice given large doses of acetaminophen or cocaine, ascorbic acid decreased damage to the liver by about 80 percent. The authors conclude that vitamin C may be a safe and effective agent for preventing liver toxicity of some drugs. *Drug and Nutrient Interaction* 3 (January–March 1984): 33–41.

Bioflavonoids

Bioflavonoids scavenge free radicals. They also have an antibiotic-like action because of their influence on cell permeability. *Biochemical Pharmacology* 32:7 (1983): 1141–1148.

Experimental animals were given a drug to induce capillary fragility. Bioflavonoids were able to prevent this condition. *Farmaco Edizione Scientifica* 38:11 (1983): 67–72.

Bioflavonoids were effective in reducing cholesterol levels in the blood and liver in experimental animals. *Indian Journal of Experimental Biology* 19 (August 1981): 787–789.

Patients suffering from chronic venous insufficiency were treated with a combination of drugs containing bioflavonoids, which proved more effective in repairing tissue damage and alleviating symptoms. *Clinica Terapeutica* 108 (January 31, 1984): 91–98.

Bioflavonoids were shown to have pharmacological properties that may prove useful in the treatment of some connective tissue disorders including rheumatoid arthritis. *Scandinavian Journal of Rheumatism* 12 (1983): 39–42.

Many bioflavonoids have anti-inflammatory effects which are considered to be superior to that of corticosteroids because of their low toxicity. Bioflavonoids are also useful for correcting capillary permeability and fragility. *Agents and Actions* 12:3 (1982): 298–302.

Thirteen out of thirty bioflavonoids tested inhibited the enzyme responsible for cataract formation. Animal studies have suggested that bioflavonoids may be useful in the prevention of cataracts in diabetics. *Biochemical Pharmacology* 31:23 (1982): 3807–3822.

Two bioflavonoids were shown to inhibit cataract formation in humans. *Biochemical Pharmacology* 32:13 (1983): 1995–1998.

CHAPTER 21: CALCIUM

Overviews

This article discusses those who may be at risk of inadequate calcium intake from poor diet; problems with absorption and utilization such as age, physical activity, estrogen deficiency, phosphorus-calcium balance, and diets high in protein, fat, and fiber. It is suggested that calcium balance can be maintained either by estrogen replacement therapy *or* by increased calcium intake. *American Journal of Clinical Nutrition* 36 (November 1982): 986–1013.

Antacids as a Source of Calcium

Adverse effects of aluminum-containing antacids include high levels of calcium secreted in the urine, bone resorption, impairment of fluoride absorption, and phosphorus depletion—all of which may contribute to bone disease. *Gastroenterology* 76 (1979): 603–606.

Osteoporosis

Calcium supplements (1000 milligrams per day) were given to fourteen postmenopausal women. The results of this study led the authors to conclude that calcium therapy, which has no serious side effects, decreases bone resorption in postmenopausal osteoporosis. Previous studies have shown that 1000–2500 milligrams of calcium per day reduced the incidence of vertebral fracture by 50 percent and that 1000 milligrams of calcium daily protected healthy menopausal women against osteoporosis. *American Journal of Clinical Nutrition* 39 (June 1984): 857–859.

In a study of twenty-six healthy women aged forty-seven to sixty-six, bone density increased with calcium supplementation *with or without* estrogen therapy. *New York State Journal of Medicine* 75 (1975): 326–336.

The author of this article suggests that the only rational approach to osteoporosis is prevention. Current data indicate that osteoporotic patients consume less calcium, require more dietary calcium to achieve calcium balance, lose more bone mass per day, and have lower vitamin D hormone levels than controls. According to one study, postmenopausal women with osteoporosis require 1500 milligrams per day of calcium to attain calcium balance compared to 1000 milligrams in premenopausal controls. *Nutrition Reviews* 41:3 (1983): 83–85.

Blood Pressure

This review article discusses various epidemiological and clinical studies correlating high calcium intakes with low blood pressure in men and pregnant and nonpregnant women. For example, in one clinical trial, 1000 milligrams of calcium given daily to hypertensives produced a 48 percent reduction in the systolic blood pressure. *Nutrition Reviews* 42:6 (1984): 205–213.

In a controlled, double-blind, randomized study, forty-eight hypertensives were given 1000 milligrams of calcium per day for eight weeks. Twenty-one of them (44 percent) achieved a therapeutically meaningful reduction in their blood pressure. Fourteen of the responders had previously required therapy with antihypertensive drugs to achieve a similar result. Oral calcium therapy was remarkably well tolerated. *Annals of Internal Medicine* 103:6 (1985): 825–831.

During a four-year controlled study of eighty-one women, half of them were given 1500 milligrams of calcium per day. In hypertensive women, those who took the supplement experienced a significant reduction in systolic blood pressure. In the unsupplemented women, systolic blood pressure continued to rise, even though they were given hypertensive medication. *American Journal of Clinical Nutrition* 42 (July 1985): 12–17.

In this study, the diets of over ten thousand adults were examined. Of the seventeen nutrients examined, low calcium was most consistently associated with high blood pressure. Intakes of potassium, sodium, and vitamins A and C were also lower in people with higher blood pressures, while cholesterol intake was not consistently different. The authors conclude that diets that restrict the intake of calories, sodium, or cholesterol may also reduce the intake of calcium and other nutrients which may be protective against hypertension. *Science* 224 (June 29, 1984): 1392–1398.

In this study, twelve normal men consumed a high-salt diet (6.6 grams per day) for two weeks. They experienced an increase in excretion of calcium and phosphorus; those who consumed a low-calcium diet also excreted more phosphorus. Men with the higher calcium intake had lower blood pressure. The authors suggest that sodium intake may influence blood pressure through its effects on calcium and potassium excretion, and that these effects may be more pronounced in people with low calcium intake. *American Journal of Clinical Nutrition* 41 (January 1985): 52–60.

In a review of the effect of calcium on blood pressure, the authors discuss recent findings that low sodium intake is related to high blood pressure and that the antihypertensive effect of calcium may depend on adequate salt intake. Severe sodium restriction may actually *exacerbate* high blood pressure, as well as reduce calcium intake by limiting consumption of dairy products. They suggest that calcium may be safe and effective as a treatment for both essential and pregnancy-related hypertension, and as a preventive measure. *Nutrition Reviews* 42 (June 1984): 205–213.

Cancer Prevention

This article reviews several studies of the relationship between vitamin D, calcium, and colon cancer. The incidence of colon cancer in Scandinavian countries was correlated with the intake of milk. In Southern California, where there is high sun exposure and milk is fortified with vitamin D, there was an association between high milk consumption and lowered risk of colon cancer. Yogurt has been shown to explicitly convey a colonic bacterial flora that inhibits the effects of known colonic carcinogens. *Nutrition Reviews* 43:6 (1985): 170–172.

A group of nearly two thousand men were followed for nineteen years. Those who developed colorectal cancer were found to have consumed significantly less calcium and vitamin D than those who did not. Men with the lowest intake had 2.7 times the risk of those with the highest intake. The authors conclude that both vitamin D and calcium may have anticancer activity. *The Lancet* I (February 9, 1985): 307–309.

Calcium Intake and Absorption

In an article that considers the nature and current implications of paleolithic nutrition, the authors determined that our early ancestors consumed approximately 1600 milligrams of calcium per day. *The New England Journal of Medicine* 312:5 (1985): 283–289.

In this article, the author reviews factors that influence calcium intake and absorption, and may therefore contribute to the development of osteoporosis. These include age, high phosphorus intake, use of drugs such as glucocorticoids (steroids), diuretics, tetracycline, and aluminum-containing antacids. Depending upon age, two thirds to three fourths of U.S. females ingest less than the RDA; fully one fourth ingest less than 300 milligrams. The author notes that a large percentage of patients with osteoporosis had a calcium imbalance with a calcium intake of 800 milligrams per day, and concludes that it is clear that the RDA of 800 milligrams cannot be sufficient for the entire population. *American Journal of Clinical Nutrition* 36 (October 1982): 776–787.

In a study of ninety-eight postmenopausal women, the authors found that malabsorption of calcium was an important risk factor for osteoporosis, probably owing to the mobilization of bone to maintain blood calcium levels. *Journal of Clinical Endocrinological Metabolism* 60 (April 1985): 651–657.

Absorption of calcium is normally only 20–40 percent of intake. A vegetarian diet contains acids that may bind 360 milligrams of calcium per day. However, over 80 percent of these acids are fermented in the intestine so that much of the calcium may be released and become available for absorption. *American Journal of Clinical Nutrition* 35 (April 1982): 783–808.

Calcium absorption may be impaired in postmenopausal women owing to inadequate stomach acid. In this population, calcium citrate is better absorbed (45 percent) than calcium carbonate (5 percent) on an empty stomach. If taken with food, calcium carbonate absorption is essentially the same as in normal people (over 20 percent). *The New England Journal of Medicine* 313 (July 11, 1985): 70–73.

Calcium malabsorption was discovered and correlated with rheumatoid arthritis activity in twenty women with this disease. Osteoporosis may result. *Annals of Rheumatoid Disease* 44 (September 1985): 585–588.

In this study, a group of women who were given 700–800 milligrams of calcium plus 375 IU of vitamin D experienced an increase in bone density. The other group of women took a balanced supplement consisting of calcium, vitamin D, and the RDA of fifteen other vitamins and minerals. This group experienced a two to three times greater increase in bone density than the other group. *Nutrition Reports International* 31 (March 1985): 741–755.

Toxicity and Adverse Effects

In a study of two hundred ulcer patients and two hundred normal controls, the authors suggest that the slightly higher risk of kidney stone formation in ulcer patients (7 versus 1 percent) was due to milk-alkali syndrome. This occurs when patients drink two to five quarts of milk per day, in addition to taking antacids. *American Journal of Gastroenterology* 68 (1977): 367–371.

CHAPTER 22: PHOSPHORUS

Overviews

This chapter discusses the uses of phosphorus in the body including its role in the bone and its many soft-tissue functions. According to the Food and Nutrition Board, the average daily intake of phosphorus is 1500–1600 milligrams. Committee on Dietary Allowances, *Recommended Daily Allowances,* ninth rev. ed. Washington, D.C.: National Academy of Sciences, 1980, pp. 133–134.

The author describes the uses of phosphorus in the body, and points out that although it is recommended that the intake of calcium and phosphorus be equal, in most diets the phosphorus intake exceeds the calcium intake. Corinne H. Robinson. *Normal and Therapeutic Nutrition*, 15th ed. New York: Macmillan, 1977, pp. 108–109.

Phosphorus/Calcium Balance

In this study, thirty-four men and women were tested for calcium and phosphorus intakes. It was found that the intakes for both minerals were higher for men than for women (1075 milligrams and 1533 milligrams versus 695 milligrams and 1095 milligrams). However, both groups were in negative balance. The authors discuss the contribution that high phosphorus intake makes to the eventual decrease in bone mass. They suggest that diets high in protein, soft drinks, and phosphorus additives are responsible for the undesirable calcium to phosphorus ratio. *American Journal of Clinical Nutrition* 40 (December 1984): 1368–1379.

CHAPTER 23: MAGNESIUM

Psychiatric Problems

Of forty-one unmedicated psychiatric patients, eleven women who attempted suicide had significantly lower cerebrospinal fluid levels of magnesium than nonsuicidal patients and controls. The authors hypothesize that magnesium may be required to maintain normal serotonergic (neurotransmitter) activity in the central nervous system. *Biological Psychiatry* 20 (February 1985): 163–171.

In this study, 165 boys who had been admitted to a psychiatric hospital were compared with normal boys. Patients with low magnesium blood levels had significantly more symptoms of depression, schizophrenia, and sleep disturbances. The authors conclude that low blood magnesium is associated with depressive and schizophrenic symptoms in children. *Biological Psychiatry* 19 (June 1984): 871–876.

The effects of vitamin B-6 and magnesium supplementation on sixty autistic children were tested in a double-blind trial. Neither supplement, when used alone, had any significant effect. A combination of the two, however, resulted in significant improvement. *Biological Psychiatry* 20 (May 1985): 467–478.

When hair samples from twenty-eight autistic children were taken, mean calcium and magnesium levels were found to be well below normal and significantly less than in controls. Although vitamin B-6 has also been found to be low in autistic children, B-6 supplementation when given without magnesium worsened the symptoms of some of the children in this study. *Orthomolecular Psychiatry* 13 (April–June 1984): 117–122.

Blood Pressure

Magnesium may modify blood pressure by interacting with other electrolytes known to affect blood vessel and smooth muscle tone, such as sodium, potassium, and calcium. *American Journal of Clinical Nutrition* 42 (1985): 1331–1338.

In this study, hypertensives had significantly less magnesium in their blood cells than did normal people. The authors point out that previous studies have shown magnesium supplementation to be an effective hypotensive agent in some types of blood pressure. *Proceedings of the National Academy of Science* 81 (October 1984): 6511–6515.

Angina

Previous studies have shown that magnesium is significantly lower in patients with angina. This study treated fifteen patients who had 5–15-minute angina attacks with intravenous magnesium. During forty-one occasions, the attacks ended within .5–2 minutes after treatment. Four patients who had daily attacks were treated daily for five days and had no further attacks. The authors contend that magnesium deficiency may be an important factor in the production of coronary vasospasm, which in turn can cause angina. *Magnesium* 3 (January–February 1984): 46–49.

Retinopathy

Eight young men with untreated hypertension and abnormal blood vessels of the retina were found to have low levels of magnesium. When supplemented with 450 milligrams of magnesium for three months, the blood vessels returned to normal. *Magnesium* 3 (May–June 1984): 159–163.

A group of seventy-one insulin-treated diabetics all had low levels of magnesium. Those with the lowest levels had the severest degree of retinal disease. The author concludes that inadequate magnesium appears to be an additional risk factor in the development and progress of this complication. *Diabetes* 27 (1978): 1075–1077.

Causes of Depletion

Magnesium deficiency results in thrombosis, and oral contraceptive use has been found to lower blood levels of magnesium. This offers a possible clue to the higher incidence of clotting disorders among women on the Pill. *Medical World News,* September 13, 1974, p. 32.

A group of "Type A" behavior men and a group of "Type B" behavior men were given a stressful task. The results of the experiment led the authors to postulate that stress causes the release of magnesium from the cells, which is then excreted in the urine. Eventual magnesium depletion can increase the risk of hypertension, coronary vasospasm (angina), and damage to the heart. *Journal of the American College of Nutrition* 4 (April–June 1985): 165–172.

The levels of magnesium in the red blood cells of women with premenstrual tension (PMT) were significantly lower than in controls. This may be due to decreased intake/absorption or increased excretion. Since PMT patients often complain of nervous tension, the magnesium may also be depleted because of stress. The author suggests that magnesium therapy may be beneficial to PMT patients with low red cell magnesium. *American Journal of Clinical Nutrition* 34 (November 1981): 2364–2366.

Magnesium in the blood serum and urine was measured in twenty-five patients who were hospitalized with Crohn's disease. Evidence of magnesium deficiency was found in 84 percent of the patients. *Journal of the American College of Nutrition* 4 (September–October 1985): 553–558.

Pregnancy Complications

In a study of 534 women with threatening premature labor, the group of patients who received magnesium supplementation experienced a reduction in the proportion of prematurity and intrauterine growth retardation. The researchers conclude that a certain percentage of these conditions are due to magnesium deficiency and can be averted with supplementation. *Magnesium* 4 (January–February 1985): 20–28.

Diarrhea

After receiving radiation therapy, twenty cervical cancer patients developed diarrhea so severe they required hospitalization. In the ten patients who were treated with magnesium, diarrhea disappeared within three days. In the group that was treated conventionally, it took two to six weeks for symptoms to clear. Radiation caused decreases in blood levels of magnesium, and the authors suggest that pretreatment with magnesium might prevent this side effect. In addition, magnesium has been found to reduce diarrhea due to malnutrition, Crohn's disease, and other conditions. *Magnesium* 4 (January–February 1985): 16–19.

Drug Interactions

Twelve bone marrow transplant patients who were treated with the drug cyclosporin experienced neurological symptoms. All patients had low magnesium levels at the onset of symptoms. These symptoms resolved or did not recur after magnesium levels were restored. The authors suggest that the neurotoxicity of this drug is due to magnesium depletion and supplementation would reduce the risk of these side effects. *The Lancet* II (November 17, 1984): 1116–1120.

CHAPTER 24: ZINC

Overviews

The authors discuss the possible symptoms of a marginal zinc deficiency in adults and children, including impaired wound healing, impaired growth, and loss of taste acuity. *Pediatric Clinics of North America* 30:3 (June 1983): 583–596.

This article reviews the possible causes of low zinc levels, including malabsorption syndromes and chronically debilitating diseases. The signs of chronic zinc deficiency include growth retardation, male hypogonadism, skin changes, poor appetite, mental lethargy, and delayed wound healing. Zinc has a wide variety of functions, including protection of the liver from carbon tetrachloride, a possible direct effect on free radicals, and the alleviation of the toxic effects of cadmium and lead. *Nutrition Reviews* 41:7 (July 1983): 206.

Absorption

Normal subjects were given zinc after an overnight fast. The absorption ranged from 40 to 86 percent. Patients with a wide variety of diseases exhibit decreased zinc absorption. *American Journal of Clinical Nutrition* 34 (1981): 2648–2652.

Three groups of healthy young men were given radiolabeled zinc after eating either 20 grams of coarse bran, Rice Krispies, or nothing. Seven days later, it was found that the group that received no food with the zinc retained the most zinc; those who ate bran absorbed the least. *Human Nutrition. Clinical Nutrition* 38C (November–December 1984): 433–441.

Laboratory rabbits were given three different forms of zinc. Zinc sulfate and zinc pantothenate appeared to be absorbed and utilized similarly. Zinc orotate was absorbed more slowly than these two. There were no significant differences in the zinc concentration in the blood. *European Journal of Drug Metabolism and Pharmacokinetics* 7:3 (1982): 233–239.

Growth and Development

Pregnant women with the lowest amount of zinc in their blood had more complications than the women with the highest amount of zinc. *American Journal of Clinical Nutrition* 40 (September 1984): 496–507.

This study found pregnant women take in marginal amounts of zinc (8.6 milligrams per day) and copper (0.95 milligrams), which results in poor body retention. Supplements containing 10–12 milligrams of zinc and 2 milligrams of copper combined with normal dietary intakes are sufficient to achieve positive balances during pregnancy. The authors point out that prenatal zinc and copper deficiencies in animals have been shown to cause birth defects. *American Journal of Clinical Nutrition* 42 (June 1985): 1184–1192.

Data show that women with zinc malabsorption and/or low blood levels of zinc have an increased risk of having a malformed child. The authors point out that few prenatal supplements contain zinc. *American Journal of Clinical Nutrition* 38 (December 1983): 943–953.

The offspring of zinc-deficient monkeys were fed a diet deficient in zinc after they were weaned. They developed bone abnormalities similar to those found in rickets. *American Journal of Clinical Nutrition* 40 (December 1984): 1203–1212.

Recent U.S. studies indicate that zinc deficiency in infants and preschool children is not uncommon. Earliest signs of deficiency include slowing of physical growth, poor appetite, and diminished taste acuity. The authors suggest that data indicate calcium carbonate in hard tap water may interfere with zinc absorption or utilization. *American Journal of Clinical Nutrition* 37 (January 1983): 37–42.

Illness, Stress, and Healing

The author notes that in many patients an upper respiratory infection with fever has been associated with a zinc deficiency. In addition, patients with severe burns have low zinc levels and severe loss of appetite, which improve with zinc supplementation. Corinne H. Robinson. *Normal and Therapeutic Nutrition*, 15th ed. New York: Macmillan, 1977, pp. 117–118.

The data from this study support other reports that injury results in zinc depletion. The average zinc levels in injured subjects in this study were significantly lower than in controls for at least four days after hospital admission. *Nutrition Research* 5 (1985): 253–261.

In an eight-week study, eighteen patients with arterial or venous leg ulcers were treated with compresses of zinc oxide. Nineteen controls were treated with unmedicated compresses. Eighty-three percent of the treated group improved, versus forty-two percent of the untreated group. Four weeks after the end of the treatment, 61 percent of the zinc oxide–treated ulcers were healed compared with 2 percent of the placebo group. The authors note that previous studies have shown that zinc given orally for one to two months improves the healing of similar ulcers in patients with low zinc levels. *British Journal of Dermatology* 111 (October 1984): 461–468.

The authors review the effectiveness of topical zinc applications in treating types 1 and 2 herpes virus lesions. Solutions of zinc have been shown to relieve pain, tingling, burning, and itching, to shorten healing time by 40–60 percent, and to reduce recurrence rates from 100 percent in controls to 0–14 percent in treated patients. For facial and upper body skin infections and genital infections, solutions can be applied as warm rinses, wet dressings, douches, or wet vaginal sponges. For oral lesions and colds due to nasal herpes, lozenges can be used. *Medical Hypotheses* 17 (June 1985): 157–165.

In a study of twenty "Type A" personalities and nineteen "Type B" personalities, the "Type A" personalities had higher levels of zinc in their red blood cells and lower levels in their urine. After a twenty-minute stressful task, urinary zinc was increased in both groups, but moreso in the "Type A." "Type A" personalities appear to deplete zinc most rapidly in stressful situations. *Journal of the American College of Nutrition* 4 (April–June 1985): 165–172.

In a study of nine healthy male runners, it was found that strenuous running led to significant losses of chromium and zinc. *Biological Trace Element Research* 6 (1984): 327–336.

Behavioral Changes

Experimental monkeys were marginally deprived of zinc from conception and compared with controls. In the deprived monkeys, the amount and variety of behavior was significantly less than the controls (10–71 percent). These and other results suggest that syndromes of lethargy, apathy, and slowed activity are characteristic behavioral effects of marginal zinc deprivation in primates. *American Journal of Clinical Nutrition* 42 (1985): 1229–1239.

Lead and Cadmium Accumulation

In a study comparing the hair mineral concentrations of normal and hypertensive women, researchers found hypertensives had 5 times as much cadmium, 2.5 times as much lead, and almost 3 times as much zinc. They suggest that enhanced dietary zinc might prevent the hypertensive effect of cadmium. *Bulletin of Environmental Contamination and Toxicology* 32 (May 1984): 525–532.

Immunity

Eighty-three normal human subjects were given 660 milligrams of zinc sulfate daily for one month. When compared to twenty untreated controls, the zinc-supplemented group experienced significantly increased lymphocyte responses. This beneficial effect does not result from a correction of latent zinc deficiency. The authors note that the supplementation of an excess of zinc had no effect on serum copper. They suggest that since the treatment is so well documented, non-toxic, and inexpensive, their findings encourage additional studies in various conditions associated with immune deficiencies. *American Journal of Clinical Nutrition* 34 (1981): 88–93.

Zinc deficiencies in animals have been shown to impair a variety of immune functions and defense mechanisms, including function of the thymus, spleen, and lymph nodes; depressed killer cells; and antibody responsiveness. These were corrected by zinc supplementation. *American Journal of Clinical Nutrition* (Supplement) 35:2 (1982): 449–451.

The author notes that zinc deficiencies have been reported in many malignant conditions, and that this is frequently associated with a high copper-to-zinc ratio. A significant survival advantage was demonstrated for patients with squamous cell lung cancer who had high zinc concentrations in their blood. *Progress in Clinical and Biological Research* 129 (1983): 1–33.

The authors studied eighty-eight healthy people aged one month to eighty-five years and seventy-two people with Down's syndrome aged ten days to twenty-five years. They found that biologically active thymic hormone (involved in immunity) decreased with age in normal subjects, and was low in most Down's syndrome subjects, regardless of age. When zinc was added to samples of their blood plasma, thymic hormone activity increased to levels found in healthy young people. *The Lancet* I (May 5, 1984): 983–986.

In a study involving kidney disease patients, the authors found that supplementation with zinc improved their lymphocyte function. *Nephron* 40 (May 1985): 13–21.

The author proposes that zinc deficiency may be a factor in the development of AIDS (Acquired Immune Deficiency Syndrome). Zinc deficiency has been associated with acquired immune deficiency states of other types; since semen contains a remarkable quantity of zinc, sexually overactive men will have a large loss of zinc. *Journal of the American Medical Association* 252 (September 21, 1984): 1401–1410.

Anorexia Nervosa

The authors studied eight women with anorexia nervosa and eight healthy women. Zinc levels after meals were significantly lower in anorexic women than in the controls. The authors hypothesize that food restriction may lead to reduced zinc levels, which in turn may result in impaired small intestinal metabolism and zinc absorption. *The Lancet* I (May 4, 1985): 1041–1042 (letter).

In this case history, a thirteen-year-old girl with anorexia nervosa was found to have an impaired sense of taste, which is a common early symptom of zinc deficiency. She was given a total of 30 milligrams of zinc per day for two weeks, and then 150 milligrams daily for four months. She regained her appetite and sense of taste and overcame her depression. Ten months after zinc supplements were stopped, she showed signs of recurrence. When supplements were resumed, she returned to normal. *The Lancet* II (August 11, 1984): 350.

Taste, Vision, and Smell

There is strong evidence to support the connection between zinc depletion and the development of night blindness and loss of taste acuity. It is likely that impaired color discrimination and smell acuity may also develop. Other investigators have suggested that such impairments may be better indicators of zinc depletion than the traditional blood tests, which are notoriously unreliable. *Annals of Internal Medicine* 99 (1983): 227–239.

The highest concentration of zinc in the human body is in the eye. It is well established that it is an essential component of the eye including the retina, choroid, cornea, and lens. Zinc deficiency causes functional impairment in various parts of the eye and there is a growing body of evidence that it is related to many conditions such as night blindness, cataract formation, and optic neuritis. *Survey of Ophthalmology* 27:2 (September–October 1982): 114–122.

The authors treated twelve chronic hemodialysis patients with zinc. Sensitivity to four taste qualities was significantly heightened, and the authors suggest that zinc replacement may be an effective therapy for loss of taste acuity in dialysis patients. *Kidney International* 24: Supplement 16 (December 1983): S315–S318.

Intake and Depletion

The authors surveyed fifty-eight people over sixty-two years of age and found that average zinc intake was only 7 milligrams (less than half the RDA). Lower taste acuity was also found in these patients, which is a symptom of zinc deficiency. These findings indicate that this population is at risk for zinc deficiency. *Journal of the American Dietetic Association* 82 (February 1983): 148–153.

The author studied forty geriatric patients, twenty of whom had senile purpura. The mean plasma level of the patients with purpura was below the lowest zinc level in the patients without this condition. The author concludes that senile purpura may be due to a zinc deficiency, possibly combined with deficiencies in other trace minerals. *Journal of Clinical Pathology* 38 (1985): 1189–1191.

The authors note that recent "advances" in food production and an increase in the consumption of highly refined foods have led to a reduction of zinc and other important nutrients. They further note that nutritional deficiency states for some of these trace elements have been reported in certain population groups. *British Journal of Nutrition* 48 (1982): 241–248.

Certain diuretics used to control hypertension cause increased zinc excretion, which may lead to zinc deficiency. Side effects of these drugs, such as impotence, may be linked to zinc depletion rather than the drugs themselves. Diuretic therapy before or after myocardial infarction may contribute to a zinc deficiency, which might slow the healing of the heart. *South African Medical Journal* 64 (December 1983): 936–941.

Zinc levels were low and prolactin levels were high in thirty-two men with end-stage kidney disease who had been undergoing hemodialysis. Zinc has been shown to inhibit prolactin synthesis *in vitro*. Zinc deficiency may be the cause of high prolactin levels in these patients. *The Lancet* II (October 5, 1985): 750–751.

Zinc deficiency has been found in people with malabsorption syndromes such as Crohn's disease, celiac disease, short bowel syndrome, and jejunoileal bypass. Diarrhea is a symptom of zinc deficiency and can also cause zinc losses. Subtle signs of zinc deficiency such as loss of appetite, impaired night vision, and depressed immune and mental functions may appear in these patients. *Journal of the American College of Nutrition* 4 (January–March 1985): 49–64.

Zinc levels in the blood were significantly lower in fifty-four patients with Crohn's disease than in nineteen healthy control subjects. The more severe the disease, the lower the levels. The authors conclude that high disease activity leads to deficiencies of zinc and that supplementation may be beneficial. *Hepatogastroenterology* 32 (January–February 1985): 34–38.

In this study, healthy men given 400 micrograms of folic acid daily excreted more zinc and had lower blood levels of zinc than controls. The authors express concern that women treated with folic acid to reverse cervical dysplasia (see Chapter 16, "Folic Acid") could develop zinc deficiency. This may be a hazard especially for users of oral contraceptives, which decrease folic acid and zinc. The authors recommend that people receiving folic acid supplements be monitored for zinc status. *Journal of the National Cancer Institute* 74 (January 1985): 263 (letter).

When blood samples from 450 pregnant women were tested, it was found that women with the lowest amount of zinc had significantly higher pregnancy complications including infection and miscarriage than those with the highest zinc. *American Journal of Clinical Nutrition* 40 (September 1984): 496–507.

Toxicity and Adverse Effects

A fifty-seven-year-old man who had been taking 450 milligrams of zinc a day for two years developed severe anemia, which appears to have been caused by impaired copper metabolism. *Annals of Internal Medicine* 103 (September 1985): 385–386.

Nine healthy young men were fed a high-protein diet which was supplemented with copper sulfate and various amounts of zinc. Based on the results of this study, the authors conclude that short-term daily intake of 18.5 milligrams of zinc resulted in increased copper excretion. *American Journal of Clinical Nutrition* 41 (February 1985): 285–292.

In a study of twenty-five men, the group that received 50 milligrams of zinc per day for six weeks did not have their blood levels of copper affected. Copper and zinc superoxide dismutase levels did decrease, which may suggest that zinc supplements decreased copper status. *American Journal of Clinical Nutrition* 40 (October 1984): 743–746.

The authors studied eleven men who were given 150 milligrams of zinc twice a day. None of the subjects showed evidence of untoward side effects. However, there was impairment of some immune functions, which returned to normal when supplements were stopped. There was also a significant decrease of HDL and a slight increase in LDL levels. *Journal of the American Medical Association* 252 (September 21, 1984): 1443–1446.

The authors gave twenty-three healthy men 50 milligrams of zinc per day for six weeks along with a diet marginal in copper. During this time, diastolic blood pressure decreased, and there was a tendency for cholesterol to decrease and HDL cholesterol to increase. *Nutrition Reports International* 32 (August 1985): 373–382.

In a study involving 270 healthy elderly people taking a zinc supplement, it appeared the zinc abolished the beneficial effects of exercise on increasing serum HDL cholesterol. *Metabolism* 34 (June 1985): 519–523.

Over 200 milligrams per day of zinc were given to two patients with Wilson's disease accompanied by severe neurological symptoms. After two years of the zinc treatment, liver copper content was reduced by 40 percent in one patient and 57 percent in the other. Their neurological symptoms almost completely disappeared. The authors note that there were no side effects in these patients, nor in others taking zinc for up to twenty-five years. *British Medical Journal* 289 (August 4, 1984): 273–276.

CHAPTER 25: IRON

Fatigue and Behavioral Changes

A double-blind study on iron therapy was conducted in chronically fatigued nonanemic women. The researchers found that there is a possibility that some chronically fatigued women may be suffering from iron deficiency even though their hemoglobin value is within the accepted normal range. These patients' individual norm for hemoglobin must be above average. *Annals of Internal Medicine* 52 (1960): 378–381.

In a group of sixty-nine normal university students, iron status was significantly related to cognitive performance. *American Journal of Clinical Nutrition* 39 (1984): 105–113.

In a study of seventy-eight iron-deficient children and forty-one nonanemic children, it was found that the iron-deficient children responded to supplementation with significantly higher school achievement scores. *American Journal of Clinical Nutrition* 42 (1985): 1221–1228.

The mental development scores for anemic infants were lower than for the group of infants with no iron deficiency and lower than the group with iron deficiency but no anemia. The anemic infants improved significantly after iron supplementation in relation to mental development, cooperativeness, and attention span. Six of the iron-deficient, nonanemic infants also showed significant improvement. The authors suggest that the effect of iron deficiency on behavior may be present during mild iron deficiency and in some cases before overt anemia. *Journal of Pediatrics* 102 (April 1983): 519–522.

Immunity

Iron deficiency is one of the likeliest forms of single micronutrient deficiency to occur. Iron is one of the most important micronutrients in terms of its influence on immune system functions and on other aspects of host defense including increased susceptibility to infection, reduced white blood cell counts, and impaired antibody production. *American Journal of Clinical Nutrition* (Supplement) 35:2 (February 1982): 442–449.

Angular Cheilosis

Of 156 cases of angular cheilosis observed in a dental practice, 19.2 percent were due to iron deficiency, and only 5.8 percent to vitamin B deficiencies. In 17 of the 30 iron-deficient patients, the condition was accompanied by smooth tongue and difficulty swallowing, which represent a premalignant condition called Plummer-Vinson syndrome. *Journal of Oral Medicine* 39 (October–December 1984): 199–206

Triglycerides

In a study involving laboratory rats, the group that was iron-deficient showed liver triglyceride levels eight times as high as the iron-sufficient controls. *Journal of Nutrition* 115 (January 1985): 138–145.

Salt Craving

A hypertensive thirty-three-year-old woman had a salt craving that caused her to consume a half pound of salt per week. After treatment with large amounts of iron, her craving decreased dramatically. The authors note that pica, the compulsive consumption of particular substances, occurs in about 50 percent of iron-deficient patients, half of whom eat ice. Salt craving is recognized as a symptom of several conditions, but has not been previously reported in connection with iron deficiency. *American Journal of Kidney Diseases* 5 (January 1985): 67–68.

Low Intakes

The authors studied the diets of seventy-four female college students. Based on four-day dietary records, they found that only six of the seventy-four met the RDA for iron. *Nutritional Reports International* 31 (February 1985): 281–285.

Iron deficiency is the most common single nutrient deficiency in the world. The authors note that even in the absence of anemia, iron deficiency may have detrimental effects on behavior and learning. *The New England Journal of Medicine* 313 (November 7, 1985): 1239–1240.

The actual foods eaten by lacto-ovo vegetarian women were analyzed and it was found that their average iron intake was 11–14 milligrams per day. These women had normal hemoglobin values, and were not considered to be anemic. However, they also did not appear to have enough iron stores to cope with heavy menstrual losses or pregnancy without possible jeopardy to their iron nutritional status. *Nutrition Report International* 27 (January 1983): 199–206.

Sports Anemia

Blood tests were performed on 43 male athletes who ran 50–200 kilometers (30–125 miles) per week and on 119 men with ordinary levels of physical activity. Some of the tests indicated that the runners showed signs of anemia, but other tests showed that inadequate iron was not the cause. The authors postulate that the runners' false anemia was due to mechanical injury of red blood cells, not to decreased iron. *Acta Medica Scandinavica* 216:2 (1984): 157–164.

Toxicity

The authors studied the effect of iron supplementation on zinc status in 291 healthy infants. They found no evidence that the iron supplements compromised zinc absorption. *American Journal of Clinical Nutrition* 42 (October 1985): 683–687.

CHAPTER 26: COPPER

Immunity

Experimentally induced deficits or excesses of copper have each been reported to increase the severity of infection in laboratory animals. *American Journal of Clinical Nutrition* (Supplement) 35:2 (February 1982): 455.

Copper Compounds

Copper complexes have been shown to be effective anti-inflammatory, anti-ulcer, anticonvulsant, anticancer, and antidiabetic agents. *Biological Trace Element Research* 5 (1983): 257–273.

Copper complexes of anti-arthritic drugs are more potent as anti-inflammatory agents, less toxic than parent compounds, and have potent anti-ulcer activity. *Inflammation* 1:3 (1976): 317–331.

Copper complexes of anti-arthritic drugs are more potent than the parent drugs and are used to treat a wide range of degenerative diseases such as rheumatoid arthritis, ankylosing spondylitis, and lupus erythematosus. *Inflammation* 2:3 (1977): 217–238.

Urinary copper was measured in five patients with chorea and in twenty-two controls. In four of the chorea patients, copper was markedly depressed. When copper supplements were given to a chorea patient, her symptoms began to lessen within three weeks, and she improved steadily over the next three months. When a placebo was substituted, her shoulder and arm jerking returned within four days. The authors suggest that copper deficiency could be an underlying abnormality in some patients with chorea. *Biological Psychiatry* 19 (December 1984): 1677–1684.

Cholesterol

Copper and other trace minerals have been shown to lower cholesterol in experimental animals and humans. A copper deficiency is associated with increased cholesterol levels and the mean copper intake in U.S. diets is approximately half the RDA. Copper deficiency is suspected to occur in the U.S. population and abroad. *Federation Proceedings* 41 (September 1982): 2807–2812.

A healthy twenty-nine-year-old man was given a copper-depleting diet for 105 days. The total cholesterol in his blood plasma increased from 202 to 234 milligrams. In addition, six abnormal heartbeats were recorded near the end of depletion. When his copper was replenished over a period of thirty-nine days, his cholesterol levels returned to normal. The authors conclude that diets inadequate in copper lead to high cholesterol and abnormal ECG patterns and may be important in the development of ischemic heart disease. *Metabolism* 33 (December 1984): 1112–1118.

Pregnancy and Oral Contraceptive Use

This study found that pregnant women take in marginal amounts of zinc (8.6 milligrams per day) and copper (0.95 milligrams), which results in poor body retention. Supplements containing 10–12 milligrams of zinc and 2 milligrams of copper combined with normal dietary intakes are sufficient to achieve positive balances during pregnancy. The authors point out that prenatal zinc and copper deficiencies in animals have been shown to cause birth defects. *American Journal of Clinical Nutrition* 42 (June 1985): 1184–1192.

In 259 pregnant women being screened for fetal abnormalities, the average blood copper level was lower in pregnancies that ended in spontaneous abortion and in which fetal abnormalities were discovered. The authors suggest that decreased copper levels in the mother may be associated with the development of spontaneous abortion and neural tube defects. *Clinical Chemistry* 30 (October 1984): 1676–1677.

Blood copper levels were significantly elevated during oral contraceptive treatment in experimental monkeys. *American Journal of Clinical Nutrition* 35 (1982): 1408–1416.

Absorption/Depletion

Copper absorption was measured in patients with celiac disease (inability to digest the gluten in cereal grains) and in healthy controls. The controls absorbed 67 percent more copper than the celiac patients. The authors conclude that patients with intestinal disease have a reduced uptake of copper, zinc, and perhaps other minerals, and may have signs of deficiency. *Science of the Total Environment* 42 (March 15, 1985): 29–36.

A thirty-six-year-old woman complained of difficulty walking and had other signs of copper deficiency including anemia. After three weeks of copper therapy, her symptoms improved. She had been taking an antacid which contained aluminum, magnesium, sodium, and other oxides for six years. The authors conclude that use of antacids should be considered a risk factor for copper deficiency. *Nutrition Reviews* 42 (September 1984): 319–321.

Copper Toxicity from Tap Water

This article reports on a family in Vermont who acquired copper intoxication from drinking water from their faucet, indicating that tap water must be taken into consideration when determining copper intakes. *Pediatrics* 74:6 (1984): 1103–1106.

CHAPTER 27: MANGANESE

Overview

The author reviews the functions of manganese in the body including normal bone growth and development, enzyme activation, normal lipid metabolism, reproduction, and nerve function. Corinne H. Robinson. *Normal and Therapeutic Nutrition*, 15th ed. New York: Macmillan, 1977, pp. 119–120.

Birth Defects

A total of sixty-one infants and their mothers were tested for manganese. Infants with congenital malformations (including central nervous system defects, cleft lip and palate, and hermaphroditism) and their mothers both had much lower levels of manganese than normal infants and their mothers. The authors conclude that low levels of manganese could be a factor in the development of birth defects. *American Journal of Clinical Nutrition* 41 (May 1985): 1042–1044.

Congenital dislocation of the hip is high in certain areas of France, Canada, and the United States. It may be due to manganese deficiency which results from the practice of alkalinizing the soil, thereby impairing the absorption of manganese by plants. Further experimental work showed that a manganese-deficient diet leads to bone and joint malformation of the offspring. *South African Medical Journal* 63:12 (1983): 393.

Epilepsy

In this study, blood manganese levels were measured in 197 young patients with convulsive disorders and 120 children without neurologic problems. The blood manganese levels were significantly lower in patients with convulsive disorders when compared to controls. The researchers conclude that low manganese levels may heighten a tendency to seizures. They also note that rats fed manganese-deficient diets have an increased susceptibility to convulsions. *Biochemical Medicine* 33 (March–April 1985): 246–255.

Immune System

Manganese stimulates microphage, phagocyte, granulocyte, and antibody activity. *American Journal of Clinical Nutrition* (Supplement) 35:2 (February 1982): 456.

Manganese deficiency reduces superoxide dismutase, a substance which prevents free radical damage. *Journal of Nutrition* 114 (1984): 1438–1446.

Glucose Tolerance

The offspring of manganese-deficient laboratory rats were maintained on a manganese-deficient diet. They experienced significantly greater hyperglycemia and lower blood insulin levels than rats fed a diet sufficient in manganese. The authors conclude that manganese deficiency during prenatal and postnatal periods may result in an impaired ability to synthesize insulin. *Journal of Nutrition* 114 (August 1984): 1438–1446.

Guinea pigs born to manganese-deficient mothers and fed manganese-deficient diets had abnormal glucose tolerance. *Journal of Nutrition* 94 (1968): 89–94.

The authors report about an eighteen-year-old male who had been controlling his diabetes with an alfalfa extract, which is high in manganese. When the hospital allowed this man to use his extract, it was found that his blood sugar could be reduced from 648 milligrams per milliliter to 68 milligrams per milliliter within two hours. This was repeated on twelve occasions, with the same response. The authors suggest that the manganese contained in the extract was responsible for the blood sugar–lowering effect. *The Lancet,* December 29, 1962, p. 1318.

Toxicity

Toxicity to manganese may occur with environmental exposure such as mining. Toxicity may appear as delusional thinking and hyperactivity. Subsequently symptoms similar to Parkinson's disease appear. *Environmental Research* 34 (1984): 242–249.

CHAPTER 28: CHROMIUM

Glucose Tolerance

In a double-blind crossover study, seventy-six volunteers were given 200 micrograms chromium per day. The researchers noted significant improvements in the glucose tolerance of a number of subjects. The authors point out that marginal dietary intake of chromium apparently is widespread in the United States and other developed countries and that often well-balanced meals do not provide adequate chromium. *American Journal of Clinical Nutrition* 36 (December 1982): 1184–1193.

Five hyperglycemic people were given 218 micrograms of chromium daily for six months. All of them had improved blood glucose control. They also had significant lowering of total serum to HDL cholesterol ratios, corresponding to halving their risk of coronary heart disease. *Nutrition Report International* 30 (October 1984): 911–918.

Six non-insulin-dependent diabetics were given approximately 20 micrograms of chromium daily in the form of brewer's yeast. After two weeks of supplementation, their mean fasting serum glucose and insulin resistance were both closer to normal. The authors postulate that chromium replenished the cells' stores of chromium and increased the effects of insulin. *General Pharmacology* 15 (November–December 1984): 535–539.

Glucose-intolerant monkeys deficient in chromium were supplemented with chromium. Some improvement was seen after three weeks; after twenty-two weeks on chromium, eight of nine previously impaired animals had normal test results. This report also cites data that demonstrate that chromium-deficient rats are less responsive to insulin than are rats given sufficient chromium. More than half of the

185 chromium-deficient rats showed a positive test for urine sugar, compared with only nine of eighty-seven chromium-supplemented controls. *Physiological Reviews* 49 (April 1969): 165–203.

Ten elderly people were supplemented with chromium. Four out of the ten experienced a disappearance of all abnormal features of the glucose tolerance test. The pattern of response in these individuals suggests the possibility that the nonresponders were suffering from such a severe chromium deficiency that a longer period of supplementation may have been required for them to have shown a response. *Metabolism* 17 (February 1968): 114–125.

High Cholesterol

This report reviews several animal and human studies that show a correlation between chromium deficiency and diabetes as well as high cholesterol levels in the blood. *Southern Medical Journal* 70 (December 1977): 1449–1453.

In this study, subjects were given 24–48 micrograms of GTF (organic) chromium, in the form of brewer's yeast, daily for eight weeks. The treatment resulted in decreased levels of total cholesterol and increased levels of HDL cholesterol. The authors found it striking that treatment with organic chromium raised HDL cholesterol in physically active, relatively young adults with normal blood lipid levels, as well as in subjects with high blood lipid levels. They also note that previous investigations have shown that GTF chromium influenced blood glucose levels, insulin response, and lipid levels. *Journal of the American College of Nutrition* 1 (1982): 263–274.

Chromium Levels in the Body

A sizable portion of the American subjects studied had low or negligible amounts of chromium in their tissues compared to individuals in other countries. The total amounts indicated that Africans had 1.9 times, Near Easterners 4.4 times, and Far Easterners 5 times as much chromium as did Americans. In addition, the aortas of American subjects showed less chromium than did those of other White, Negro, and Oriental subjects from around the world. *American Journal of Clinical Nutrition* 21 (March 1968): 230–244.

Marginal dietary chromium intake is widespread in the United States and other developed countries. In a double-blind study of seventy-six people, chromium or a placebo was given for three months. Chromium was used as well as absorbed by the subjects, as indicated by a significant improvement in the glucose tolerance of a number of subjects. *American Journal of Clinical Nutrition* 36 (December 1982): 1184–1193.

In a study of nine healthy male runners, the authors found that strenuous running led to significant losses of chromium, presumably because of its increased use in glucose metabolism. *Biological Trace Element Research* 6 (1984): 327–336.

CHAPTER 29: SELENIUM

Absorption/Intake/Requirements

According to this study, selenium levels were significantly greater in humans with selenomethionine than with a selenite supplement. *American Journal of Clinical Nutrition* 42 (1985): 439–448.

Forty-six alcoholics were compared with forty-five nonalcoholic individuals. Alcoholics had low blood selenium levels, especially if their livers were diseased. The authors conclude that inadequate selenium intake is likely in alcoholics; impaired absorption, increased requirements, or altered metabolism of selenium may also be factors. Selenium deficiency, by reducing glutathione peroxidase activity, may contribute to liver damage in alcoholics. *American Journal of Clinical Nutrition* 42 (July 1985): 147–151.

In this study, thirty young women were given 150 micrograms of sodium selenate per day, 600 milligrams of vitamin C per day, or both. After four weeks, selenium levels were increased by 34 percent in the women taking selenium only, by 29 percent in those taking vitamin C only, and by 63 percent in those taking both. The authors conclude that vitamin C improves the bioavailability of dietary selenium. *Human Nutrition. Clinical Nutrition* 39C (May–June 1985): 221–226.

The authors found that TPN (total parenteral nutrition) patients have lower blood levels of selenium and vitamin E, and recommend supplementation with these nutrients in these individuals. *American Journal of Clinical Nutrition* 42 (1985): 432–438.

Blood selenium levels were measured in sixteen patients with celiac disease and thirty-two healthy controls. Selenium levels in plasma, leucocytes, and whole blood were significantly lower in celiac patients than in the controls. The authors hypothesize that gluten-free diets might be deficient in selenium, or that selenium may be poorly absorbed by celiac patients. Decreased selenium levels in these individuals may explain the increased incidence of cancers of the gastrointestinal tract and other parts of the body which has been reported in celiac patients. *British Medical Journal* 288 (June 23, 1984): 1862–1863.

The authors studied twenty-three patients with Down's syndrome and found significantly lower plasma selenium levels than in controls. They encourage further studies including a trial of selenium supplementation. *Acta Paediatrica Scandinavica* 73 (1984): 275–277.

The authors studied eighty-six Texas oil refinery workers. Selenium levels were significantly lower in industrial workers than in controls. Their glutathione peroxidase levels were also lower. The authors conclude that lower selenium was not due to dietary inadequacy, but may be due to exposure to environmental oxidants that may affect selenium status. *Nutrition Research* 3 (1983): 805–817.

There is a continuing, but controversial interest in the use of hair as a diagnostic tool for the assessment of trace element status. The authors of this paper studied blood and hair selenium before, during, and after selenium supplementation. Selenium supplementation for six weeks caused no increase in plasma selenium levels, but did cause an increase in selenium levels in new hair growth. There was a significant decline in hair selenium levels during the final six weeks after the selenium supplement was withdrawn. There was no correlation between hair and blood selenium levels. *Nutrition Research* 4 (1984): 577–582.

Cancer

The authors review the anticancer properties of selenium in humans and experimental animals. Dietary selenium intake is inversely correlated with death from leukemia and cancers of the breast, ovary, lung, colon, rectum, and prostate. Selenium should be considered not only as a preventive, but also as a therapeutic agent in cancer treatment and may act additively or synergistically with drug and X-ray treatments. *Journal of Agricultural Food Chemistry* 32 (May–June 1984): 436–442.

Many animal studies demonstrate a cancer-protective effect of selenium. Human epidemiological studies suggest that cancer risk is reduced in people living in high selenium areas, in people with high selenium food supply, and in people with higher blood levels of selenium. *Seminars in Oncology* 10 (September 1983): 305–310.

Selenium supplementation in animals reduces the frequency of chemically induced cancers and inhibits the growth of transplanted tumors. In a study of over 10,000 people, the average selenium level of 111 subjects who subsequently developed cancer was lower than that of the 210 matched controls. Also, the risk of cancer was twice as high for people in the lowest quintile of selenium levels. *The Lancet*, July 16, 1983, pp. 130–134.

In this study involving 240 patients with skin cancer and 103 controls, the mean selenium level for all skin cancer patients was significantly lower than control values. This study therefore supports the hypothesis that higher blood selenium levels reduce the risk of developing some cancers. *Nutrition and Cancer* 6 (January–March 1984): 13–21.

A population of over 8000 with low selenium levels was followed for six years. Cancer was subsequently diagnosed in 128 people, who had significantly lower selenium levels than the controls. The authors suggest that selenium may act by reducing the mutagenicity of carcinogens, by affecting carcinogen metabolism, or by protecting against oxidative damage. *American Journal of Epidemiology* 120 (September 1984): 342–349.

The authors studied 12,000 people in Finland, 51 of whom died of cancer during the following four years. They found that selenium levels were significantly lower in cancer patients than in controls, and the difference was greater in smokers than in nonsmokers. The risk of cancer mortality in people with the lowest selenium levels was nearly six times greater than that of controls. For people with both low selenium levels and low vitamin E levels, the risk of death from cancer was more than eleven times that of people who had higher levels of both these nutrients. The data suggest that dietary selenium deficiency is associated with an increased risk of fatal cancer, that low vitamin E intake may enhance this effect, and that decreased vitamin A intake contributes to the risk of lung cancer among smoking men with low selenium intake. *British Medical Journal* 290 (February 9, 1985): 417–420.

This study showed that vitamin E enhances selenium's ability to inhibit the development of breast cancer in laboratory rats treated with a potent carcinogen. In general, the chemopreventive effect of selenium is manifested in the form of lower tumor incidence, a reduction in the size of tumors, and a longer latency period. *Cancer Research* 43 (November 1983): 5335–5341.

The combined effect of selenium and vitamin A on breast cancer development in rats was studied. This investigation provided evidence that vitamin A increases the protective effect of selenium, and the authors suggest that the results warrant further study. *Cancer Research* 41 (April 1981): 1413–1416.

Several geographic studies have suggested that states or countries with higher selenium levels in the soil and in locally grown food experience lower death rates from cancer. The author of this review article found that the results of such studies indicate a decreased mortality from cancer of the lung, colon, rectum, bladder, esophagus, pancreas, breast, ovary, and cervix. Lower selenium levels have been found in patients with various types of cancer, as well as lower levels of vitamins E and A and beta-carotene. The author emphasizes the need to consider several nutrients in diet and cancer studies, instead of focusing on just one nutrient per study. He also points out that current selenium trials are limited to 200 micrograms per day, which may not be the optimum amount needed to prevent cancer. *Federation Proceedings* 44 (June 1985): 2584–2589.

In a study of 1458 healthy adults in twenty-four regions of China, low blood selenium levels were associated with higher deaths from cancer of the stomach, esophagus, liver, and all sites. The authors expect that selenium supplementation will reduce cancer incidence. *Biological Trace Element Research* 7 (January–February 1985): 21–29.

Immunity

Selenium is needed for a fully functioning immune system. Studies with mice have shown that the offspring of selenium-deficient mice had impaired immune responses, and that selenium supplements enhanced the effects of vaccines. When a modest excess of selenium was given to dogs, it stimulated their immune systems. This effect was greatest when they were fed diets high in polyunsaturated fats. *American Journal of Clinical Nutrition* (Supplement) 35:2 (1982): 452–453.

Heart Disease

The authors studied over 8000 people in Finland. During a follow-up period of seven years, 367 of these people had a heart attack or died of heart disease. Their mean serum selenium levels were lower than controls. Those with the lowest selenium levels had a six to sevenfold increase in the risk of death from heart disease. *The Lancet*, July 24, 1982, pp. 175–179.

Muscular Dystrophy

The author notes that it is well known that muscular dystrophy in cattle and sheep is a selenium-deficiency disease preventable by giving selenium to these animals. In this study of twenty-four patients with muscular dystrophy, serum selenium levels were lower for patients than controls. Patients who were more severely disabled had lower selenium levels than patients with mild symptoms. One patient received selenium therapy and experienced considerable functional improvement. The authors suggest that muscular dystrophy may be a selenium deficiency disease. A long-term study is being undertaken. *Acta Medica Scandinavica* 211 (1982): 493–499.

Rheumatoid Arthritis

The authors measured selenium levels of eighty-seven rheumatoid arthritis patients. Low selenium levels were found in all patients, with lowest levels in those with the most severe disease. Although selenium deficiency is probably not a primary etiological factor in rheumatoid arthritis, patients with low selenium levels may develop more severe disease. Selenium supplementation might have some therapeutic benefit in rheumatoid arthritis. *Scandinavian Journal of Rheumatology* 14 (April–June 1985): 97–101.

Seven rheumatoid arthritis patients who no longer responded to conventional treatment were given 350 micrograms of selenium and 400 IU of vitamin E daily. Ten to fourteen days later their normal treatment was resumed. In four patients, joint pain disappeared; in the remaining three patients, joint pain was diminished and mobility was markedly increased. *Biological Trace Element Research* 7 (May–June 1985): 195–198.

Skin Conditions

In a study of patients with acne, those given selenium (400 micrograms per day) and vitamin E (25 IU per day) showed improvement in their condition. In patients not treated, there was a marked worsening of the acne. A few patients who were previously treated with zinc and tetracycline experienced complete healing of the acne when given the supplements. In addition, three patients with seborrheic dermatitis also improved with this treatment. *Acta Dermatologica Venerealogica* 64 (1984): 9–14.

Mental Well-Being

In a double-blind study involving thirty elderly people, half received 1720 micrograms of sodium selenate, 45 micrograms of organic selenium, and 400 milligrams of vitamin E; the other half received a placebo. After two months, the supplemented group showed obvious improvement in mental well-being when compared with controls. They showed significant improvement in fatigue, anorexia, depression, anxiety, emotional lability, hostility, mental alertness, motivation and initiative, self-care, and interest in the environment. There were no adverse effects after one year of treatment. *Biological Trace Element Research* 7 (April–May 1985): 161–168.

Toxicity

The authors report the average daily intake in an area which was high on selenium but free of toxicity was 750 micrograms. The authors indicate that the chronically toxic dose of dietary selenium is likely to be near 5 milligrams (5000 micrograms) per day. The chronically toxic dose of sodium selenate is estimated to be lower, in the range of 1 milligram per day. *American Journal of Clinical Nutrition* 37 (May 1983): 872.

The authors review numerous data on the toxicity of selenium. Various studies have shown no adverse effects from the long-term consumption of 500 micrograms, 350 micrograms, or 600 micrograms daily. Selenium intake in China is reported to be 750 micrograms per day with no signs of toxicity. Toxicity for selenium, extrapolated from animal studies, may occur in humans ingesting 1000–2000 micrograms per day. The Food and Nutrition Board has stated that toxicity occurs in humans ingesting 2400–3000 micrograms daily. Based on these data, they point out the board's claim that the safe upper limit is 200 micrograms per day is a conservative one and has definite implications for chemoprevention studies based on supplementation. *Seminars in Oncology* 10:3 (1983): 311–319.

CHAPTER 30: IODINE

Overview

The author reviews the functions of iodine, dietary sources, and geographical regions of high incidence of iodine deficiency. Corinne H. Robinson. *Normal and Therapeutic Nutrition.* 15th ed. New York: Macmillan, 1977, pp. 115–116.

Thyroid

Iodine in the form of sodium iodide can be used to treat goiter and hyperthyroidism. A severe iodine deficiency can cause hypothyroidism. *The Merck Manual,* 14th ed. Rahway, N.J.: Merck Sharp and Dohme Research Laboratories, 1982, pp. 997–1012.

Hearing

Children in an area of China with endemic iodine deficiency had a lower hearing level than children in an area without endemic iodine deficiency. After three years of iodine supplementation, thyroid function tests and hearing levels became normal. The authors suggest that hearing loss is one of the iodine deficiency disorders that are now being identified based on a broader understanding of iodine deficiency states. *The Lancet,* September 7, 1985, pp. 518–520.

Nuclear Accidents

A nuclear reactor accident could pose a hazard to the public because of the release of radioactive iodine, which could damage the thyroid and ultimately lead to thyroid cancer. In the event of such an accident, a single dose of 300 milligrams of potassium iodide would block the uptake of radioactive iodine by the thyroid, and may be advisable in high-risk individuals. *The Lancet,* February 1983, p. 451.

It is believed that predistribution of potassium iodide tablets to households near nuclear power plants may be worthwhile as a preventive measure in the event of a nuclear accident. *Public Health Reports* 98 (April 1983): 123–126.

CHAPTER 31: POTASSIUM

Overview

The author reviews the uses of potassium in the body, good dietary sources, and the causes and symptoms of deficiency. Corinne H. Robinson. *Normal and Therapeutic Nutrition,* 15th ed. New York: Macmillan, 1977, pp. 130–131.

Bioavailability and Retention

Since many potassium chloride supplements are distasteful, many physicians tell their patients to consume large amounts of potassium-rich foods, usually in the form of fruit. The authors measured the potassium levels in various fruits and concluded that the retention of potassium in these foods is poor. The authors conclude that potassium chloride supplements must continue to be the mainstays for potassium repletion. *The New England Journal of Medicine* 313 (August 29, 1985): 582–583.

Increasing potassium and decreasing sodium in diets could benefit people with hypertension, those who are overweight, and some diabetics. The authors suggest several approaches to achieving a more favorable sodium-to-potassium ratio in the diet: preserving potassium through steaming rather than boiling foods; adding modest amounts of potassium chloride salt substitute to cooking water; and adding less salt. *The Lancet*, February 12, 1983, pp. 362–363.

Blood Pressure

The authors studied the relationship between dietary nutrients and blood pressure in over ten thousand people. The 10 percent of the group with the highest blood pressure tended to have decreased intakes of calcium, potassium, vitamin A, and vitamin C. *Science* 224 (June 29, 1984): 1392–1398.

Only 2 percent of vegetarians have been found to have high blood pressure, as compared with 26 percent of nonvegetarians. Vegetarians with the highest potassium excretion, indicating a high intake, had the lowest blood pressure. *American Journal of Clinical Nutrition* 37 (May 1983): 755–762.

The authors of this article studied twelve subjects with mild hypertension. Some subjects responded to sodium restriction while others responded to potassium supplementation. The authors conclude that individuals respond differently to changes in sodium or potassium intake. *The Lancet*, April 7, 1984, pp. 757–761.

Hypertensive Kidney Damage

Salt-sensitive rats fed a high-salt diet developed hypertension and related symptoms. When potassium was added to their diet, blood pressure was unchanged, but there was less damage to the kidneys. The authors suggest that potassium exerts a protective effect and that blacks in the United States, who have a low potassium intake and a high rate of hypertensive kidney failure, might benefit from tripling their potassium intake. *Hypertension* (Supplement I) 6 (March–April 1984): 1170–1176.

Stroke

Hypertensive, stroke-prone rats were fed a stroke-inducing diet. After six weeks, the group supplemented with potassium had a systolic blood pressure of 187, versus 233 for the unsupplemented group. After seventeen weeks, death (due mainly to strokes) was 2 percent in the supplemented group, versus 83 percent in the controls. Mortality was seven times greater in the unsupplemented group than in the supplemented group, even when blood pressure was the same. The authors conclude that potassium intake at levels similar to those in prehistoric human diets (6–10 grams per day) may reduce stroke incidence even when blood pressure is not lowered. *Hypertension* (Supplement I) 7 (May–June 1985): I110–I114.

INDEX

individual ODA programs, 33, 34, 35, 36, 37, 38, 39, 41, 42; intake and absorption of, 207–8; and magnesium, 60, 120–21, 126, 128–29; major uses, 167; ODA, 120–21, 167; and phosphorus, 118, 121–22, 123, 124, 125, 209; RDA, 118–19; supplements, kinds, 116, 121–22; toxicity and adverse effects of, 122, 208

Calcium ascorbate, 109

Calcium bicarbonate, zinc and, 133

Calcium pantothenate, 98

Calories (calorie intake), 16–17; daily menus and, 48–50; RDAs and, 16–17; "well-balanced diet" and, 16–17

Cancer (carcinogens), 3, 4, 9, 19, 21, 25; A and beta-carotene and, 29, 32, 33, 56–57, 58, 59, 153, 178–79, 228; aging and, 21; B-1 and, 77, 186; B-2 and, 79; B-3 and, 83, 189; B-6 and, 88; B-12 and, 195; C and, 9, 19, 27, 30, 32, 34, 92, 104, 105–6, 108, 200; calcium and, 4, 60, 181, 207; causes, 50–51; copper and, 142, 221; cruciferous vegetables and, 47; D and, 60, 181; diet and, 50; E and selenium and, 3, 4, 27, 32, 64, 67, 152–54, 183, 226, 227–28; folic acid and, 94, 196–97; free radicals and, 26 (see also Free radicals); individual ODA programs and, 32, 33–34; lifestyles and, 50; manganese and, 145, 146; nitrosamines and, 19 (see also Nitrosamines); RDAs and, 19, 21; zinc and, 32, 132, 214–15. See also Chemotherapy; Radiation therapy; specific kinds

Capillary fragility, bioflavonoids and, 111, 205

Carbohydrates, 16, 25, 46; B-1 and metabolism of, 76–77, 78; refined, manganese lacking in, 146; utilization, phosphorus and, 123. See also specific kinds

Carbon tetrachloride, 131

Carcinogens. See Cancer (carcinogens)

Cardiovascular system and problems, 25, 27, 32; B-6 and, 192; copper and, 142; E and, 64, 67, 182; magnesium and, 127; ODAs and, 170; potassium and, 159; selenium and, 151. See also Arteries; Coronary heart disease; Heart disease

Carpal tunnel syndrome, 74, 86–87, 89;

B-2 and, 80, 81, 87, 187–88; B-6 and, 74, 80, 86–87, 89, 191

Carrot juice, 58

Cataracts: bioflavonoids and, 111, 205; B-2 and, 79, 81, 187; E and, 63; selenium and, 151; zinc and, 132, 216

Cauliflower, 47

Caveman diet, 23, 107

Celiac disease, 20, 66, 133, 143, 152, 217, 222, 226

Cells (cellular processes): phosphorus and, 123–24; zinc and, 130. See also Tissues; specific conditions, kinds

Cereals (cereal grains), 120, 134, 139; whole grain, 47, 48, 49, 134, 143. See also Grains

Cervical dysplasia (cervical cancer): A and, 178, 179; C and, 200; folic acid and, 94–95, 96, 179, 196–97, 217; magnesium and, 211

Cheese, 48, 49, 119–20, 149, 160

Cheilosis, 80; angular, 80, 138, 219

Chelated supplements, 45

Chemical pollutants (toxic chemicals), 19, 20, 50; C and, 99; free radicals and, 26–27; selenium and, 152, 154; zinc and, 131. See also Toxins; specific kinds

Chemotherapy, 7, 33; A and, 57, 179; C and, 105; E and, 64, 183

Chicken, 48, 49, 50, 99, 134. See also Poultry

"Chinese Restaurant Syndrome" (MSG), B-6 and, 88, 194

Chocolate, 47

Cholesterol, 4, 6–7, 27, 33, 64–65, 159; biotin and, 99; B-3 and, 4, 27, 82, 189; C and, 106, 201; choline, inositol, and PABA and, 101, 199; chromium and, 148–49, 150, 225; copper and, 142, 221; E and, 4, 64–65; HDLs and LDLs (good and bad), 4, 7, 27, 64–65, 82, 106, 135–36, 142, 149, 199, 201, 218; lecithin and, 101, 199; Questran and, 21; zinc and, 135–36, 218

Choline, 72, 101, 102, 103, 199; cautions, 103; food sources, 102, 166; ODA, 102, 166; supplements, forms, 102

Chorea, 142, 221

Chromium, 14, 40, 148–50, 224–26; food sources, 149–50, 168; individual programs and GTF, 33, 34, 35, 36, 37, 38, 39, 40 (see also GTF); major uses